Canolol and Derivatives

As the demand for natural and sustainable solutions grows, *Canolol and Derivatives: Chemistry, Extraction, Properties and Application in Food* explores the science and potential of canolol, a powerful antioxidant derived from oilseed products like canola and mustard. With antioxidant activity surpassing compounds like vitamin C and quercetin, canolol offers exceptional promise for food preservation and health applications, including anti-inflammatory, anticancer, and antimutagenic benefits.

KEY FEATURES:

- Canolol's unique chemistry and formation during oilseed processing
- Advanced extraction technologies, including green and sustainable methods
- Its role as a natural alternative to synthetic antioxidants like BHA and BHT
- Applications in food preservation, nutraceuticals, and therapeutic uses

Essential for researchers, food scientists, and industry professionals, this book provides the knowledge to unlock canolol's potential as a transformative natural antioxidant and health-promoting agent.

Canolol and Derivatives
Chemistry, Extraction, Properties and Application in Food

Edited by

Michael N. A. Eskin and Bertrand Matthäus

CRC Press
Taylor & Francis Group
Boca Raton London New York

CRC Press is an imprint of the
Taylor & Francis Group, an **informa** business

Designed cover image: Shutterstock

First edition published 2026
by CRC Press
2385 NW Executive Center Drive, Suite 320, Boca Raton FL 33431

and by CRC Press
4 Park Square, Milton Park, Abingdon, Oxon, OX14 4RN

CRC Press is an imprint of Taylor & Francis Group, LLC

ISBN: 978-1-032-25034-2 (hbk)
ISBN: 978-1-032-25035-9 (pbk)
ISBN: 978-1-003-28122-1 (ebk)

DOI: 10.1201/b22828

Typeset in Palatino
by SPi Technologies India Pvt Ltd (Straive)

Contents

Preface

With this book we want to summarize the knowledge about an important antioxidant compound formed during the processing of canola oil. Canolol or 4-vinylsyringol is a unique phenolic compound first discovered in crude canola oil. It is not naturally occurring but formed by decarboxylation of sinapic acid at elevated temperatures during the pressing or roasting of canola seeds. Sinapic acid is derived from sinapine, the choline ester of sinapic acid, which is the predominant phenolic compound present. Sinapic acid is the major free phenolic compound in canola and rapeseed, accounting for 70.2–85.4% of free phenolic acids in the defatted seeds. Removal of choline from sinapine leads to the formation of sinapic acid, which can be converted to canolol by heat or sinapic acid decarboxylase. In addition to canola, mustard and hemp seeds are also rich sources of sinapic acid and potential sources of canolol.

This book provides detailed coverage of canolol and its properties. Chapter 1 is a brief introduction to the discovery and formation of canolol, while Chapter 2 is an extensive review of the green methods available for generating and extracting canolol. The qualitative and quantitative methods for measuring canolol are presented in Chapter 3. The bioproduction of canolol from canola meal feedstock using an engineered sinapic acid decarboxylase is described in detail in Chapter 4. The powerful antioxidant properties of canolol are discussed extensively in Chapter 5, while the anti-cancer properties of canolol are reviewed in Chapter 6. The final chapter, Chapter 7, covers the important applications of canolol in enhancing the stability of foods and beverages as well as reducing waste.

The idea for this book came from our colleague and friend, the late Usha Thiyam-Hollander, who tragically passed away from cancer in 2020, just prior to the beginning of the pandemic. Our aim was to finalize her idea and publish a book about this interesting natural compound and therefore we are extremely grateful for the important contributions to this book by outstanding scientists from around the world. This book provides an up-to-date coverage of canolol as an effective antioxidant and anticancer agent. We would like to acknowledge the excellent editorial assistance provided by Taylor & Francis.

Michael N. A. Eskin
Bertrand Matthäus

About the editors

Dr. Michael N. A. Eskin, a former Chair and Associate Dean, is a Distinguished Professor in the Department of Food and Human Nutritional Sciences in the Faculty of Agricultural and Food Sciences at the University of Manitoba, Winnipeg, Canada. He is the author and co-author of 20 books, 80 chapters, and over 170 papers. Dr. Eskin is the recipient of many prestigious awards for his lipid research, including the Stephen S. Chang Award and the Lifetime Achievement Award in Honor of Nicolas Appert by the Institute of Food Technologists; the Supelco AOCS Research Award, Stephen S. Chang Award, Alton E. Bailey Medal, Herbert J. Dutton Award, Timothy L. Mounts Award and Distinguished Service Award by the American Oil Chemists' Society; and the William J. Eva Award by the Canadian Institute of Food Science and Technology. In 2016, Dr. Eskin was awarded the Order of Canada for his significant contributions to the success of the Canadian canola oil industry and recently inducted into the Canadian Agricultural Hall of Fame.

Dr. Bertrand Matthäus, heads since 2021 the Department of Safety and Quality of Cereals at the Max Rubner-Institut, Federal Research Institute of Nutrition and Food of the German Federal Ministry of Agriculture, Nutrition, and Regional Identity. During his career he has been responsible for research regarding improvements in the quality of fats and oils, especially canola oil. His work focused on the investigation of frying processes but included also contaminants such as 3-MCPD ester, acrylamide or 4-hydroxy-2-trans-nonenal, and the investigation of oxidation processes of edible oils and fats. He has published over 200 articles, scientific papers, and book chapters. In the last 25 years he has organized and co-organized several symposia and workshops on fats and oils given for official laboratories, private institutions, and industry. He is vice-president of the German Society for Fat Science, and he has been awarded the prestigious Wilhelm Normann Medal in 2019 for his work on edible fats and oils. In 2024, he was awarded the "Bianzhong Award" of the Hubei Provincial Government. He is the co-author with Dr. Michael N. A. Eskin and the late Dr. Usha Thiyam-Hollander of *Canola and Rapeseed: Production, Processing, Food Quality, and Nutrition.*

Contributors

Ewa Bąkowska
Department of Food Biochemistry and Analysis
Poznań University of Life Sciences
Poznań, Poland

Krzysztof Dwiecki
Department of Food Biochemistry and Analysis
Poznań University of Life Sciences
Poznań, Poland

Michael N. A. Eskin
Department of Food & Human Nutritional Sciences
University of Manitoba
Winnipeg, Manitoba, Canada

Olamide Fadairo
Department of Food and Human Nutritional Sciences
University of Manitoba
Winnipeg, Manitoba, Canada

Richardson Centre for Functional Foods & Nutraceuticals
Winnipeg, Manitoba, Canada

Supratim Ghosh
Department of Food and Bioproduct Sciences
College of Agriculture and Bioresources
University of Saskatchewan
Saskatoon, Canada

Bertrand Matthäus
Department of Safety and Quality of Cereals
Max Rubner-Institut, Federal Research Institut for Nutrition and Food
Detmold, Germany

Krista L. Morley
Aquatic and Crop Resource Development Centre
National Research Council of Canada
Montréal, Quebec, Canada

Ruchira Nandasiri
Department of Food and Human Nutritional Sciences
University of Manitoba
Winnipeg, Manitoba, Canada

Richardson Centre for Functional Foods & Nutraceuticals
Winnipeg, Manitoba, Canada

St. Boniface Albrechtsen Research Centre
Winnipeg, Manitoba, Canada

Maryam Nikbakht Nasrabadi
Department of Food and Bioproduct Sciences
College of Agriculture and Bioresources
University of Saskatchewan
Saskatoon, Canada

Aleksander Siger
Department of Food Biochemistry and Analysis
Poznań University of Life Sciences
Poznań, Poland

Karin Schwarz
Institute of Human Nutrition and Food Science
Division of Food Technology
Kiel University
Kiel, Germany

Xia Xiang
Oil Crops Research Institute
Chinese Academy of Agricultural Sciences. Oil Crops and Lipids Process Technology National & Local Joint Engineering Laboratory, Key Laboratory of Oilseeds Processing, Ministry of Agriculture and Rural Affairs, Hubei Key Laboratory of Lipid Chemistry and Nutrition
Wuhan, China

Zhenxia Xu
Oil Crops Research Institute
Chinese Academy of Agricultural Sciences, Oil Crops and Lipids Process Technology National & Local Joint Engineering Laboratory, Key Laboratory of Oilseeds Processing, Ministry of Agriculture and Rural Affairs, Hubei Key Laboratory of Lipid Chemistry and Nutrition
Wuhan, China

chapter one

Canolol: Introduction

Michael N. A. Eskin and Bertrand Matthäus

Canola and low erucic acid rapeseed are among the richest sources of polyphenols compared to other oilseeds (Di Lena et al., 2021; Wongsirchot et al., 2022). The corresponding meals, by-products of oil refining, are rich sources of hydroxycinnamic acids, primarily sinapic acid esters. Sinapine (sinapoyl choline), in particular, accounts for over 80% of the total phenolic compounds present in the meal. Besides the meal, phenolics such as canolol (4-vinyl-2,6-dimethoxy-phenol) were first reported by Koski et al. (2003) in rapeseed oil at elevated temperatures and confirmed later by Wakamatsu et al. (2005) (Figure 1.1).

Harbaum-Piayda et al. (2010) subsequently identified canolol in the deodistillates produced during the refining of rapeseed oil. The formation of canolol is closely associated with the Maillard reaction products where carbohydrates and proteins interact with phenolic compounds producing different protein-phenol and carbohydrate-phenol complexes when subjected to high temperatures and pressures (Keyhani & Yaylayan, 2002).

It was also reported that formation of canolol takes place during high pressure and temperature processing and is not found naturally in the sample matrix (Li & Guo, 2016; Nandasiri et al., 2019, 2021a). The formation of canolol from sinapine involves two steps. First is the loss of choline from sinapine to form sinapic acid (Nandasiri et al., 2019). The latter then undergoes decarboxylation with the formation of canolol.

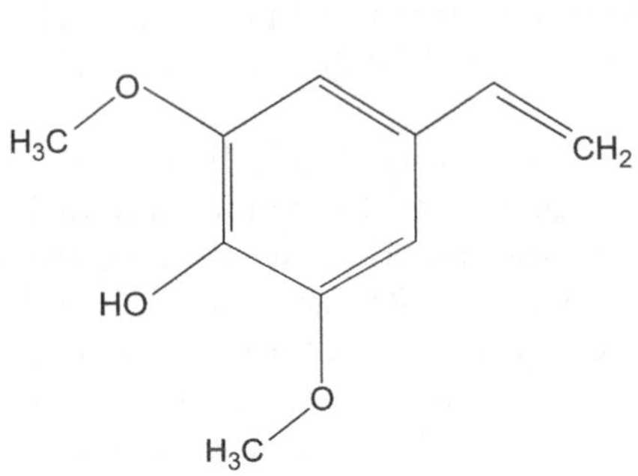

Figure 1.1 The chemical structure of canolol.

DOI: 10.1201/b22828-1

Other rich plant sources of sinapic acid include hemp and yellow mustard (Zago et al., 2022; Nguyen et al., 2023). It was further observed that these matrixes including mustard (both oil and meal) was able to generate canolol at high temperatures (>140°C) (Thiyam-Hollander et al., 2014) and pH adjustments (6.5–8.5) (Nguyen et al., 2023). An engineered sinapic acid decarboxylase was also shown to produce canolol from sinapic acid (Morley et al., 2013). Other methods include the synthesis of canolol from syringaldehyde by Wittig olefination in hexane/tetrahydrofuran (THF) or condensation of syringaldehyde and malonic acid using microwave irradiation (Figure 1.2).

The production of canolol from the meal fraction of rapeseed/canola has been studied using a variety of pretreatments and extraction techniques including enzymes, microwave, and air frying (Zago et al., 2015; Fadairo et al., 2022; Nandasiri et al. 2023). A previous study by Nandasiri et al. (2021b) reported a unique solvent-free green pretreatment using a modified RapidOxy®100 equipment combined with ultrasound assisted extraction. Using this system they effectively enhanced the production of canolol from canola meal. Yu and co-workers (2020) subjected rapeseed to a steam explosion pretreatment which resulted in the production of rapeseed oil with superhigh canolol content.

In general, the concentration of canolol was comparatively higher in the oil fraction than the meal, implying its lipophilic nature and hydrophobicity (Thiyam-Hollander et al., 2014; Kraljić et al., 2015). However, with the application of pressurized temperature processing canolol was extracted in water extracts by reducing the surface tension and thereby improving the hydrophilicity (Li & Guo, 2016; Nandasiri et al., 2019). The presence of ester bonds and a hydroxyl group at the para position along with a double bond attached to the ortho position makes canolol a highly reactive compound (Gaspar et al., 2009). Due to its high reactivity it converts into other forms including dimers, trimers, and oligomers at elevated temperatures (Harbaum-Piayda et al., 2010; Kraljić et al., 2015; Nandasiri et al., 2021a). Further, it was observed that formation of canolol is highly correlated to its initial free sinapic acid (before roasting) (0.94) and residual sinapic acid (after roasting) (0.98) content in high erucic mustard seeds (Shrestha et al., 2012).

High reactivity of canolol is closely linked to its structure with the double bonds. In the presence of oxygen, canolol is oxidized and converts into different forms including its dimers, trimers, and oligomers (Harbaum-Piayda et al., 2010; Kraljić et al., 2015). Hence, extraction of canolol in an enclosed system therefore is desirable to prevent any further oxidative losses (Nandasiri et al., 2019). The increased antioxidant activity and the higher radical scavenging activity of canolol accommodate its suitability in both food and oil systems as a natural preservative

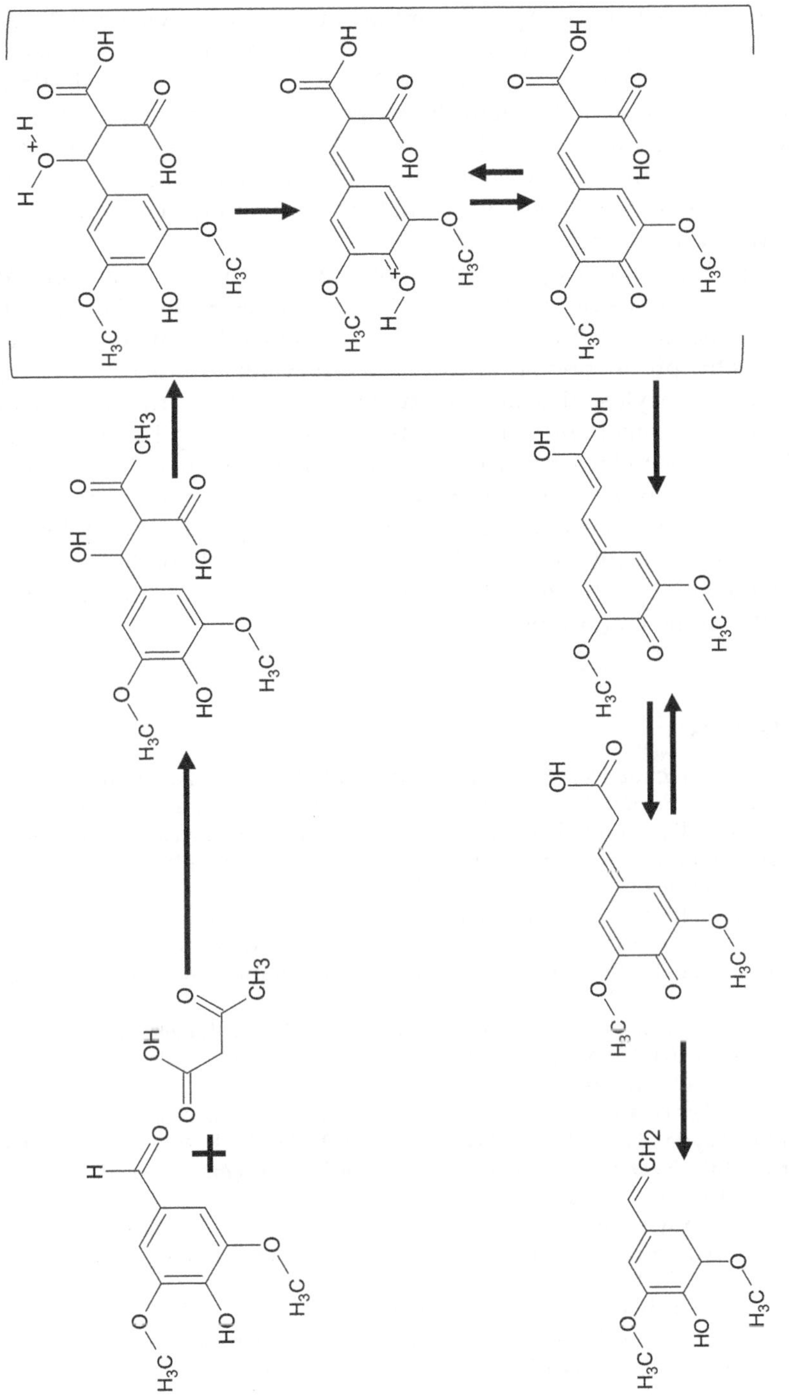

Figure 1.2 Synthesis of canolol from syringaldehyde (Shrestha et al., 2012).

elongating the shelf-life. Apart from the antioxidant activity, canolol also exhibited many anti-mutagenic properties with potential applications in human health (Nandasiri & Eskin 2022). Advancements in application of natural products in food systems have opened up a wide area of study for including canolol as a natural antioxidant compound. Hence, this book encloses the detailed analysis of canolol as a potential antioxidative, antimicrobial, and natural preservative in both food and feed systems and its respective health benefits.

Chapter 2 covers optimization of the extraction of canolol from canola/rapeseed using green technology. Chapter 3 describes the analytical methods used for analyzing canolol and its derivatives. Chapter 4 discusses the production of canolol from renewable resources using engineered decarboxylase. The latter enzyme catalyzes the formation of canolol from sinapic acid and was the subject of a review by Lamiscolo et al. (2023). This was followed by the identification of new phenolic acid decarboxylase in the brown-rot fungus *Neolentinus lepideus* capable of producing canolol. The strong antioxidant and anticancer properties exhibited by canolol make it a suitable bioactive for use in the food and health-related industries. Finally, Chapter 7 discusses a number of potential applications of canolol in the food industry.

References

Di Lena, G., Sanchez Del Pulgar, J., Lucarini, M., Durazzo, A., Ondrejickova, P., Oanca, F., Frincu, R.M., Aguzzi, A., Ferrari Nicolli, S., Casin, I., Gabrielli, P., Caproni, R., Cerven, I., Lombardi-Boccia, G. (2021) Valorization potentials of rapeseed meal in a biorefinery perspective: Focus on nutritional and bioactive components. *Molecules* 26, 6787.

Fadairo, O.S., Nandasiri, R., Nguyen, T., Eskin, N.A.M., Aluko, R.E., Scanlon, M.G. (2022). Improved extraction efficiency and antioxidant activity of defatted canola meal extract phenolic compounds obtained from air-fried seeds. *Antioxidants* 1, 2411.

Gaspar, A., Garrido, E.M., Esteves, M., Quezada, E., Milhazes, N., Garrido, J., Borges, F. (2009). New insights into the antioxidant activity of hydroxycinnamic acids: Synthesis and physicochemical characterization of novel halogenated derivatives. *European Journal of Medicinal Chemistry* 44, 2092–2099.

Harbaum-Piayda, B., Oehlke, K., Sönnichsen, F.D., Zacchi, P., Eggers, R., Schwarz, K. (2010). New polyphenolic compounds in commercial deodistillate and rapeseed oils. *Food Chemistry* 123, 607–615.

Keyhani, A., Yaylayan, V.A. (2002). Glycine specific novel maillard reaction products: 5-Hydroxy-1,3-dimethyl-2(1 H)-quinoxalinone and Related Compounds. *Journal of Agricultural and Food Chemistry* 45, 697–702.

Koski, A., Pekkarinen, S., Hopia, A., Wahala, K., Heinonen, M. (2003). Processing of rapeseed oil: Effects on sinapic acid derivative content and oxidative stability. *European Food Research and Technology* 217, 110–114.

Kraljić, K., Škevin, D., Barišić, L., Kovačević, M., Obranović, M., Jurčević, I. (2015). Changes in 4-vinylsyringol and other phenolics during rapeseed oil refining. *Food Chemistry* 187, 236–242.

Lamiscolo, A., Odinot, E., Villeneuve, P., Lecome, J. (2023). Challenges and advances in biotechnological approaches for the synthesis of canolol and other vinylphenols from biobased *p*-hydroxycinnamic acids: A review. *Biotechnology for Biofuels and Bioproducts* 16, 573.

Li, J., Guo, Z. (2016). Concurrent extraction and transformation of bioactive phenolic compounds from rapeseed meal using pressurized solvent extraction system. *Industrial Crops and Products* 94, 152–159.

Morley, K.L., Grosse, S., Leisch, H., Lau, P.C.K. (2013). Antioxidant canolol production from a renewable feedstock via an engineered decarboxylase. *Green Chemistry* 15(112), 3312–3317.

Nandasiri, R., Eskin, N.A.M. (2022). Canolol and its derivatives: A novel bioactive with antioxidant and anticancer properties. *Advanced Food and Nutrition Research* 100, 109–129.

Nandasiri, R., Eskin, N.A.M., Komatsu, E., Perreault, H., Thiyam-Holländer, U. (2021a). Valorization of canola by-products: Concomitance of flavor-active bitter phenolics using pressurized heat treatments. *LWT* 138, 110397.

Nandasiri, R., Eskin, N.A.M., Thiyam-Höllander, U. (2019). Antioxidative polyphenols of canola meal extracted by high pressure: Impact of temperature and solvents. *Journal of Food Science* 84, 3117–3128.

Nandasiri, R., Fadairo, O., Nguyen, T., Zago, E., Anas, M.U.M., Eskin, N.A.M. (2023). Optimization of canolol production from canola meal using microwave digestion as a pre-treatment method. *Foods* 12(2), 318.

Nandasiri, R., Imran, A., Thiyam-Holländer, U., Eskin, N.A.M. (2021b). Rapidoxy® 100: A solvent-free pre-treatment for production of canolol. *Frontiers in Nutrition* 8, 687851.

Nguyen, T., Nanadasiri, R., Olamide, F., Eskin, N.A.M. (2023). The effect of pH on the phenolic content and antioxidant properties of three different mustard extracts. *Journal of Food Science*, 88, 2882–2901.

Shrestha, K., Stevens, C.V., Meulenaer, B. De. (2012). Isolation and identification of a potent radical scavenger (canolol) from roasted high erucic mustard seed oil from Nepal and its formation during roasting. *Journal of Agricultural and Food Chemistry*, 60, 7506–7512.

Thiyam-Holllander, U., Aladedunye, F., Logan, A., Yang, H., Diehl, B. (2014). Identification and quantification of canolol and related sinapate precursors in Indian mustard oils and Canadian mustard products. *European Journal of Lipid Science and Technology*, 116, 1664–1674.

Wakamatsu, D., Morimura, S., Sawa, T., Kida, K., Nakae, C., Maeda, H. (2005). Isolation, identification, and structure of a potent alkyl-peroxyl radical scavenger in crude canola oil, canolol. *Bioscience Biotechnology and Biochemistry* 69, 1568–1574.

Wongsirchot, P., Gonzalez-Michel, M., Winterburn, J. (2022). Recent advances in rapeseed meal as alternative feedstock for industrial biotechnology. *Biochemical Engineering Journal* 180, 108373.

Yu, G. Guo, T., Huang, Q. (2020). Preparation of rapeseed with superhigh canolol content and superior quality characteristics by steam explosion pretreatment technology. *Food Science and Nutrition* 9, 2271–2278.

Zago, E., Lecomte, J., Baarouh, N., Aouf, C., Carre, P., Fine, F., Villeneuve, P. (2015). Influence of rapeseed meal treatments on its total phenolic content and composition in sinapine, sinapic acid and canolol. *Industrial Crop Production* 76, 1061–1070.

Zago, E., Nandasiri, R., Thiyam-Hollander, U., Eskin, N.A.M. (2022). Influence of thermal treatments ion the antioxidant activity of hemp cake polar extracts. *Journal of Food Science and Technology* 59, 3256–3265.

chapter two

Extraction and production of canolol: Application of green technology

Ruchira Nandasiri, Olamide Fadairo, and Michael N. A. Eskin

2.1 Introduction

Over the years the importance of natural antioxidant compounds has risen due to the implications of synthetic antioxidant compounds including BHA and BHT. The food industry is currently looking for alternative options for natural preservatives and antioxidant compounds as shelf-life enhancers. Hence, the oilseed industry is specifically looking for natural antioxidants to limit lipid peroxidation (Harbaum-Piayda et al., 2010; Nandasiri et al., 2019). Until now, natural antioxidant compounds have been successful but rosemary extracts can impart flavor and aroma to the final product (Khattab et al., 2014). Canolol recently has gained the attention of researchers due to its higher antioxidant potential and antiradical activity (Nandasiri & Eskin, 2022). Canolol is not a natural phenolic compound and is generated during thermal processing at high temperatures and pressure via the conversion of sinapine and sinapic acid (Khattab et al., 2014; Nandasiri et al., 2019).

The importance of canolol has risen over the years due to its strong radical potential (Kraljić et al., 2019). Canolol was first discovered in canola oil processed under higher temperatures (Harbaum-Piayda et al., 2010). It was found that during the refining and deodorization stages of the oil extraction oxidative stability of the oils was not impacted due to the formation of canolol in canola oil (Harbaum-Piayda et al., 2010). Later it was discovered that not only canola but also mustard has the same trend in the formation of canolol (Thiyam-Holländer et al., 2014). Later it was also discovered that the formation of canolol not only takes place through the thermal processing of oil but also with the by-product meal (Khattab et al., 2014; Nandasiri et al., 2019). Both canola and mustard by-products demonstrated that the formation of canolol takes place with extensive thermal processing (Fadairo et al., 2021; Nandasiri et al., 2019; Nandasiri et al.,

DOI: 10.1201/b22828-2

2021a, 2021b, 2021c). It was later observed that alterations in the processing conditions including temperature, pressure, and pH could impact the formation of canolol (Fadairo et al., 2021; Nandasiri et al., 2019; Nandasiri et al., 2021a, 2021b, 2021c; Nguyen et al., 2023). The concentration of canolol was comparatively higher in the oil fraction than in the meal (Fadairo et al., 2022). The higher availability of canolol in oil fractions further suggests that canolol is lipophilic in nature and in stable lipid fractions (Kuwahara et al., 2004). The oilseed industry is one of North America's leading industries, making a significant contribution to its economy. Both canola and mustard industries primarily focus on increasing their yield and improving their quality (Kuwahara et al., 2004).

The use of excessive solvents and electricity during the processing operations of the oilseed industry has major effects on the environment. As many industries are currently trying to reduce their carbon footprint, alternative green extraction techniques with less or no solvent use toward oilseed processing are favored. Many modern oil refining facilities are designed to produce high-quality stable oils, therefore, the majority of the minor components are removed during their processing steps (Eskin, 2020). Hence, natural antioxidant compounds like canolol could withstand these extreme processing conditions while adding value to the oils. Extreme pressure and temperature conditions applied during the oilseed processing operations favor the conversion of sinapine to sinapic acid and canolol via hydrolysis and decarboxylation (Khattab et al., 2013; Nandasiri et al., 2019).

However, due to the presence of ester bonds and a hydroxyl group at the para position and a double bond attached to the ortho position makes canolol a highly reactive substance to oxygen and could easily oxidize. During the oxidation process of canolol its structure could alter to create many different forms of dimers, trimers, and oligomers (Harbaum-Piayda et al., 2010; Kraljić et al., 2015; Nandasiri et al., 2021a). Consequently, an enclosed system is preferred for the extraction of canolol. Although it demonstrates high antioxidant activity, extraction of canolol has not been studied extensively up to date. The current chapter will discuss the possibility of application of green and environmentally friendly extraction techniques to extract canolol from both oil and meal fractions.

2.2 Canolol

2.2.1 The structure, chemistry, and synthesis

Canolol (2,6-dimethoxy-4-vinylphenol/4-vinylsyringol) (Figure 2.1) is a derivative of sinapic acid. The IUPAC name of canolol is 4-ethenyl-2,6-dimethoxyphenol. Structurally, canolol contains two esters, a hydroxyl group at the para position, and a double bond attached to a phenyl group.

The molecular formula of canolol is $C_{10}H_{12}O_3$ and it has a molecular mass of 180.203 $gmol^{-1}$ as well as a monoisotopic mass of 180.078644

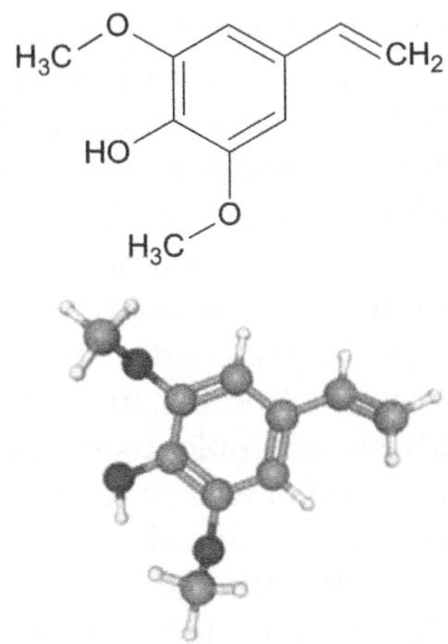

Figure 2.1 The chemical structure of canolol.

gmol^{-1}. According to its structure it has a hydrogen bond donor count of one and acceptor count of three. The different active groups present in canolol make it highly reactive and provide strong antioxidant potential. In addition, it has a topological polar surface area of 38.7 Å^2. The European Union has categorized canolol into the food additive class as a flavoring agent in regulation (EU) No 872/2012.

As mentioned earlier, canolol is not a naturally occurring compound and is synthesized by a decarboxylation reaction of sinapic acid (Figure 2.2). Canolol is the predominant sinapic acid derivative detectable in rapeseed oil relative to other phenolic derivatives (1.6–17.06 mg/100 g). Significant variations in the quantity of these phenolic compounds in rape seed are attributed to factors such as agronomy, environmental, genetic, and production procedures (Yang et al., 2014). The formation of canolol

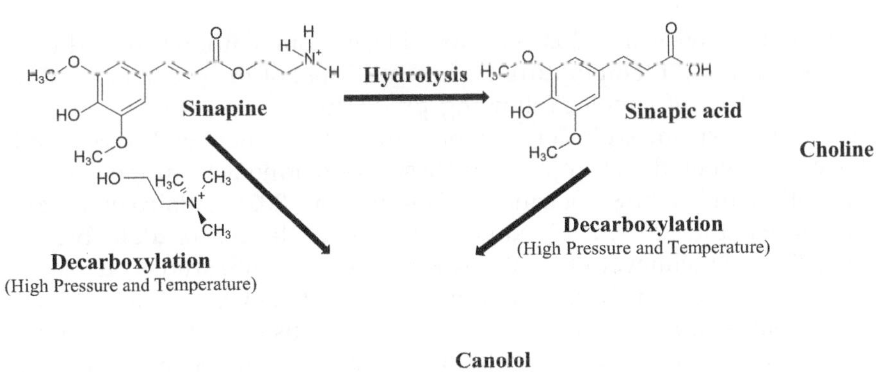

Figure 2.2 Formation of canolol from sinapine and sinapic acid.

is a two-step process which involves sinapine being hydrolyzed first into sinapic acid, then followed by the decarboxylation of sinapic acid into canolol (Thiyam et al., 2009). Another instance also found direct conversion of sinapine into canolol via the decarboxylation (Figure 2.2). Syringic acid also can be used to chemically synthesize the canolol. The other methods include the condensation of syringaldehyde and malonic acid using microwave irradiation (Figure 2.3). Through a series of chain reactions in the presence of piperidine, syringaldehyde can be converted into canolol in the presence of microwave radiation. Khattab et al. (2013) also conducted a study on chemical synthesis of canolol using the microwave technology. In their study, formation of canolol was done using microwave radiation of sinapic acid in the presence of 1,8-diazabicyclo [5.4.0] undec-7-ene (DBU) with aluminum oxide and hydroquinone.

Khattab et al. (2013) further reported that conversion of sinapic acid to canolol was over 50% with the current microwave extraction method. As the formation of canolol under high temperature and pressure could be categorized into a Maillard type reaction, the Maillard reaction products of different protein-phenol and carbohydrate-phenol complexes could be formed during the formation of canolol (Keyhani & Yaylayan, 2002). The lower conversion rates of sinapic acid to canolol can be attributed to this phenomenon. In addition to the traditional chemical extraction techniques, green extraction methods including enzymatic hydrolysis and the novel application of ultrasound, and microwave-aided solvent extraction and solvent-free pretreatment methods including air-frying and modified RapidOxy® method were used to produce canolol from both oil and the by-product meal (Cao et al., 2019; Nandasiri et al., 2021b). In addition, significant variations in the quantity of canolol in rapeseed and canola are attributed to factors such as agronomy, environmental, genetic, and production procedures (Yang et al., 2014).

2.2.2 Stability

Canolol (4-vinylsyringol) is very unstable at room temperature and when subjected to high temperature treatments. Most of the previous work on the formation of canolol following pre-treatment operations, including dry heating, steam explosion, and pressurized treatment of Brassica seeds, have documented the impacts of these pretreatment techniques on the formation and stability of canolol (Fadairo et al., 2021; Fadairo et al., 2022; Nandasiri et al., 2019, 2023; Nandasiri et al., 2021a, 2021b, 2021c; Nguyen et al., 2023; Spielmeyer et al., 2009). Kraljić et al. (2015) studied the stability of canolol under three conditions: freezing (–20°C), cooling (4°C), and room temperatures (20 to 25°C). The authors observed that canolol was most stable under freezing condition with 20% of canolol lost after five (5) months. In contrast, canolol was quite unstable and the degradation rate was quite rapid at 4°C with about 50% loss, while at room temperature there was complete breakdown with no canolol detected after five months.

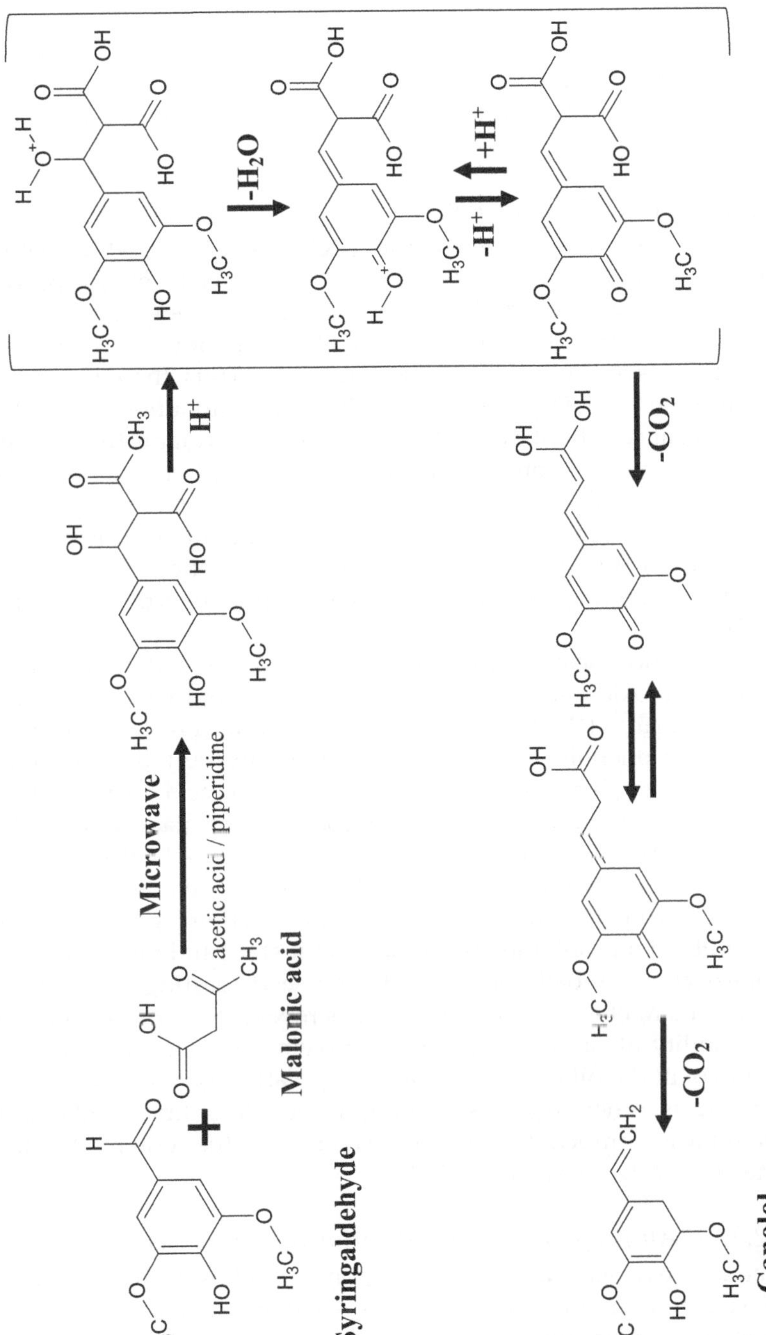

Figure 2.3 Synthesis of canolol from syringaldehyde. **(Adapted from Shrestha et al. 2012).**

2.2.3 *Bioactivity*

Phenolic compounds are phytochemicals essential for the biological functions of the plant. It is well established that hydroxycinnamic acids exhibit strong antioxidative properties by scavenging free radicals (Teixeira et al., 2013).

2.2.3.1 *Antioxidant activity*

Antioxidants are reactive oxygen species (ROS) scavengers, which help to maintain the concentration of ROS in the body at a given level by capturing the excess (Murtaza et al., 2013). Under normal physiological condition, the endogenous antioxidants may not be able to maintain this balance, leading to the onset of various disease conditions. Thus, there is need for the consumption of dietary antioxidant phenolic compounds to maintain the delicate balance. Attention has been given to antioxidants from natural sources. The increasing concern by consumers to replace synthetic antioxidants with natural antioxidants in their food products suggests that canolol would conform to this "clean label" requirement. Canolol as a sinapic acid derivative is receiving considerable attention because of its antioxidative, antimutagenic, and anticarcinogenic properties (Nandasiri & Eskin, 2022).

The free-radical scavenging efficacy of canolol is better than many well-known antioxidants, such as quercetin, α-tocopherol, vitamin C, β-carotene, and rutin (Wakamatsu et al., 2005). The antioxidant activity of sinapate-related phenolic compounds decreased in the following order: canolol derivatives (dimer/trimer) > canolol > sinapic acid > sinapoyl glucose > sinapine (Thiyam et al., 2006). According to Galano et al. (2011), the biological activity of canolol, such as its powerful radical-scavenging capacity and reactivity with peroxide radicals, was essentially due to the transfer of a hydrogen atom from the phenolic functional group. The oxidative stability of oils obtained from roasted mustard and rapeseed is due to the presence of canolol generated during seed roasting (Koski et al., 2003; Wijesundera et al., 2008). Some studies revealed an improvement in the heat stability of canola oil when deep-frying by increasing the content of canolol in the oil (Aachary et al., 2014; Matthäus et al., 2014). Using accelerated tests, other studies showed that the rate of lipid oxidation in rapeseed oil was significantly delayed by increasing the content of canolol (Shrestha et al., 2012; Zhang et al., 2014).

2.2.3.2 *Anti-inflammatory and anti-carcinogenic activity*

Inflammation represents a defensive response of a host to contagion and tissue destruction, marked by a series of reactions, such as vasodilation and engagement of immune cells and plasma proteins at the area of infection or tissue damage (Lawrence, 2009; Zhang & Sun, 2015). The nuclear factor NF-kB pathway is regarded as a classical example for the inflammation promoting and signaling pathway, largely based on the role of NF-kB in the expression of proinflammatory substances such as cytokines, chemokines, and adhesion molecules (Liu et al., 2017). NF-κB is fundamental in signaling phagocytes, in which an improper regulation of protein could lead to cancer, as well as inflammatory and autoimmune diseases (Shukla & Singh, 2011). Fang et al. (2013), demonstrated in an in-vivo study that the anti-inflammatory action of 4-vinyl-2,6-dimethoxyphenol (canolol) against bowel disease and associated colitis carcinogenesis was through obstruction of inflammatory cytokines and oxidative stress. The biological activities of canolol in the suppression of inflammation and carcinogenesis was reported by Cao et al. (2008). Furthermore, another pathway that demonstrated the antiproliferative effect of SA against the T47D cell line has been reported (Hudson et al., 2000; Kampa et al., 2003). Canolol has also been shown to be an effective and powerful, antimutagenic, anti-cancer, and antioxidant phenolic compound (Siger et al., 2017). The antioxidant and antimutagenic properties of canolol have been shown to be comparable to those of tocopherol, rutin, and quercetin, and β-carotene (Kuwahara et al., 2004; Siger et al., 2017).

2.3 *The impact of preheat treatment and frying*

Pretreatments have gained considerable attention in both the food and nutraceutical industries as a method for improving the antioxidative phenolic compounds. Among the pretreatments, heating and frying have garnered attention for phenolic antioxidants associated with oilseeds (Fadairo et al., 2021; Harbaum-Piayda et al., 2010). The formation of canolol was found to have a positive relationship with the preheat treatment temperatures (Nandasiri et al., 2019). Hence, at extreme temperatures canolol would be converted into its other forms including dimer and trimers thereby reducing its concentration (Harbaum-Piayda et al., 2010; Kraljić et al., 2015). A recent study conducted by Nandasiri et al. (2019) found that when subjected to high pressure (1500 psi) and temperatures above 160°C, the concentration of canolol decreased in the canola meal extracts obtained from 0.5 mm particle size with both 70% (v/v) ethanol (297.98 ± 51.25 μg/g DW) and 70% methanol (251.72 ± 16.80 μg/g DW), while the total phenolic, flavonoid contents and antioxidant activity increased. However, canola meal extracts obtained from the 1.0 mm particle size at extraction temperatures of 180°C showed the highest recovery of canolol for both 70% (v/v) ethanol (342.48 ± 37.83 μg/g DW) and 70% methanol (491.29 ± 42.58 μg/g DW) extractants (Nandasiri et al., 2019).

Similarly, another study conducted by Nandasiri, Imran, et al. (2021b) found that preheat treatment prior to ultrasonic extraction in canola meal samples had a similar trend toward the extraction of canolol. When canola meal was pretreated at different temperature and time combinations they found that the pretreatment temperature-time combination of 160°C for 10 min (453.40 ± 17.66 μg/g DW) and 180°C for 5 min (427.11 ± 7.12 μg/g DW) were the optimum pretreatment combinations for extracting canolol in an inert environment (Nandasiri et al., 2021b). Another study conducted by Fadairo et al. (2021) found that pretreatment temperature-time combination of 170°C for 15 min (1086.08 ± 12.62 μg CE/100g) was optimum for extracting canolol from lower-grade yellow mustard seeds after air-frying. They also found that the antioxidant activity of the extracts subjected to air-frying at both 170°C and 180°C at 15 min were higher compared to the other treatment temperature-time combinations. These novel findings open up new ways of optimizing the extractability of canolol from different oilseed varieties and its by-products. However, further investigations are required to define the optimum extractability conditions for canolol in comparison to current processing conditions.

Matthäus et al. (2014) reported that canolol-enriched extracts obtained from the super-critical carbon dioxide treatment were able to improve the frying performance of high-oleic canola oil during 30 h of deep-frying. They also reported that the oxidative stability of the oils treated with canolol-enriched extracts were higher compared to oils treated with TBHQ (200 mg/kg) and rosemary extracts (200 mg/kg) (Matthäus et al., 2014). In addition, the degradation rates of both α- and γ- tocopherols were comparatively lower in the oils treated with canolol-enriched extracts after 30 h of deep-frying. Additionally, it was also reported that canola distillate extracts were able to stabilize the oils during deep fat frying (Matthäus et al., 2014). A study conducted by Aachary et al. (2014) evaluated the oxidative stability of deep fried oils at 185°C for 5 min for 5 days with a total frying time of 6 h per day. The results indicated that the frying oil containing either a crude canolol extract or a canola oil distillates extract exhibited better oxidative stability than the frying oil containing BHT (Aachary et al., 2014). They also reported that the total oxidation (TOTOX) and conjugated diene/triene values of oils stabilized with deodistillates or crude canolol were significantly ($p<0.05$) lower than for oils containing BHT (Aachary et al., 2014).

2.4 Extraction of canolol

2.4.1 Conventional methods

Extensive research has been conducted on a number of extraction methods on various mustard fractions including seeds (Kozlowska et al., 1990), flour (Thiyam-Holländer et al., 2014), leaves (Park et al., 2014), hulls and cotyledons (Mayengbam et al., 2014), and meals (Dubie et al., 2013; Engels et al., 2012). Of the various extraction technologies, the most widely used are aqueous solutions of methanol or ethanol that may be coupled with ultrasonic treatment (Fadairo et al., 2022; Chadni et al., 2021; Nandasiri et al., 2019; Park et al., 2014; Thiyam-Holländer et al., 2014; Dubie et al., 2013; Mayengbam et al., 2014; Thiyam et al., 2004). Some authors also documented extraction methods using solvent under pressure (Kozlowska et al., 2016; Nandasiri et al., 2019), methanol-chloroform mixtures (Ishtiaque et al., 2013; Kozlowska et al., 2016) or acetone-methanol-0.1% formic acid mixtures (Engels et al., 2012). Rasera et al. (2019) investigated the optimum solvent mixture for the recovery of antioxidant compounds from two types of mustard seeds (white – *Sinapis alba* and black – *Brassica nigra*) using a simplex centroid mixture design. The authors reported that compared with pure acetone, extraction with a water-acetone solvent mixture produced a phenolic extract with a much greater antioxidant activity that showed a 48-fold increase in 2,2-azinobis-(3-ethylbenzothiazoline-6-sulfonate) ($ABTS^{\bullet+}$), a 23-fold increase in total phenolic content (TPC), and a 25-fold increase in the 2,2-diphenylpicrylhydrazyl (DPPH) values. A similar treatment of black mustard resulted in an extract with 31-, 19-, and 27-fold higher values for ABTS, TPC, and DPPH, respectively, compared to the corresponding extract with pure acetone.

From an analytical perspective with laboratory applications, solvent extraction remains the most popular method employed in the extraction of canola oil following pretreatment and/or pressing of the seeds (Bubalo et al., 2015; Kumar et al., 2017). Liquid-liquid extraction of phenolic compounds using a mixture of organic and polar solvents has received considerable attention over time. Koski et al. (2003) extracted phenolic compounds from virgin olive and rapeseed oil using an equal proportion of hexane and aqueous methanol. In other studies, by Fadairo et al. (2021) and Fadairo et al. (2023), the authors employed liquid-liquid extraction of canolol from mustard and canola oil using an equal proportion of hexane and 70% (v/v) methanol. Aqueous methanol proved to be effective for extracting phenolic compounds from oilseeds. While hexane is a very effective organic solvent, it poses significant environmental challenges (Kumar et al., 2017). Other limitations with the use of organic extractants for oil extraction are their low reproducibility, long processing times, low mass transfer, and high energy consumption (Kumar et al., 2017).

2.4.2 *Emerging green extraction methods*

Emerging concerns about sustainability of the planet has demanded the development of eco-friendly or green processing technologies for food production and manufacturing (Kumar et al., 2017). Consequently, there is a need for novel and green alternative methodologies using safe solvents capable of extracting phenolic compounds from plants, such as rapeseed and mustard. This technological shift to eco-friendly and sustainable practices must be cost effective and process efficient and provide positive benefits to consumers in terms of food safety, nutritional composition, and sensory properties. To meet consumer concerns, alternative and efficient technologies are being explored that are environmentally friendly and sustainable for the canola and mustard industries. Green chemistry is focused on reducing the use of hazardous materials by developing safer and alternative technologies (Kumar et al., 2017). A number of these alternative technologies shun the use of carbon-based solvents for the extraction of oilseeds (Dunford, 2012). These emerging pretreatment and processing techniques include the use of supercritical CO_2 extraction, micro-emulsions extraction, microwave-assisted extraction, ultrasound extraction, air-frying, Deep Eutectic Solvent (DES), Pressurized Solvent Extraction (PSE), Pulsed-Electric Field (PEF), and enzyme-assisted extraction.

Extensive studies have been conducted on the extraction, identification, and quantification of phenolic compounds in oilseeds and by-products using conventional solvents assisted with nonconventional techniques. Li and Guo (2016) investigated the simultaneous extraction and transformation of phenolics in rapeseed meal using a pressurized solvent extraction procedure. The authors reported the highest TPC of 92.53 and antioxidant activity in terms of DPPH free radical scavenging activity of 66.68 mg SAE/g rapeseed meal with aqueous methanol, temperature of 200°C, and 20 min. This was over 300% more than that obtained from Soxhlet extraction conditions (100°C for 12 h). The maximum canolol content (7.23 mg/g) was obtained with 100% methanol, 200°C, and 5 min with 1% NaOH in methanol (w/v). Khattab et al. (2014) reported the successful production of canolol from sinapine in canola meal via hydrolysis to sinapic acid and then with microwave-induced decarboxylation. The authors reported that a microwave power of 300 W for 12 min yielded the highest sinapic acid conversion to canolol (58.3 %), resulting in 4.2 mg canolol for each gram of canola meal. The extraction of phenolics is readily conducted by pure or aqueous solvents including ethanol or methanol using conventional extraction techniques. However, conventional solvents show certain drawbacks including high toxicity, non-biodegradability, high cost, low boiling points, and high flammability (Lohani et al., 2015).

2.4.2.1 *Supercritical fluid extraction*

A supercritical fluid has the typical density of a liquid, viscosity indistinguishable from that of a gas, and diffusivity in between a liquid and a gas. Supercritical fluids possess much better transport properties than liquid owing to their low viscosity and high diffusivity (Mukhopadhyay, 2000; Jenab et al., 2013). Because of their unique physicochemical properties, supercritical fluid extraction (SFE) provides several operational merits over traditional extraction methods (Wang et al., 2021). SFE offers a rapid rate of extraction and high yield, and is an eco-friendly procedure with little or no use of carbon-based solvents.

Carbon dioxide is the most popular and frequently used fluid for SFE applications due to its low critical constants (Tc=31.1°C; Pc=72.8 atm), its nontoxic and nonflammable properties, low cost, and ready availability in high purity (Wang et al., 2021). Supercritical CO_2 is an emerging "green" option for the extraction of oils and bioactive constituents with potential applications in the food, pharmaceutical, and cosmetics industries, because it is amenable to moderate pressures and temperatures (Nautiyal, 2016; Zhang et al., 2014). SC-CO_2 extraction is green and efficient, meeting the requirements of "Green Extraction" technology (Belwal et al., 2018). SC-CO_2 extraction processes can be summarized as follows: CO_2 heat exchange, CO_2 pressurization, extraction of soluble substances, separation of SC-CO_2 from extract, and recycling of the resultant CO_2 (Chemat & Vorobiev, 2019). SC-CO_2 extraction efficiency largely depends on pressure, temperature, solvent flow rate, and addition of chemical modifiers (De Melo et al., 2014; Essien et al., 2020). The major limitation of SC-CO_2 is its low polarity, and this has been successfully controlled by the addition of chemical modifiers such as ethanol and methanol. The solvent characteristic of supercritical CO_2 makes it a perfect choice for the extraction of non-polar compounds (Castro-Vargas et al., 2019; Sato et al., 2019; Tuhanioglu & Ubeyitogullari, 2022; Valadez-Carmona et al., 2018). Extensive research has been conducted on the extraction of phenolic compounds from plant matrices using SC-CO_2, with or without co-solvents. The distinctive features of SC-CO_2 allow it to be applied in extraction, particle formation, preservation, extrusion, and drying, all of which have been documented in articles and patents. Extraction is the most documented application of SC-CO_2 from plant materials, including the decaffeination of coffee and tea (Wang et al., 2021), although limited studies exist on the use of SC-CO_2 for the extraction of phenolics from canola/mustard seeds co-products. An earlier study was done by Sun et al. (2008) on the supercritical CO_2 extraction of phenolic acids from canola meals with/or without ethanol as co-solvent. The authors concluded that the phenolic acid contents of SC-CO_2-extracted meals were higher than meals extracted with SC-CO_2 with ethanol. Ferrentino et al. (2018) conducted a comparative study on the recovery of antioxidants from apple pomace using SFE and conventional extraction. The authors revealed that extracts obtained from SFE with the operating condition of 30 MPa and 45 °C for 2 h with 5% ethanol as co-solvent exhibited a better phenolic content and higher antioxidant activity (5.63 ± 0.10mgTEA/g of extract) than conventional extraction technologies, namely, Soxhlet with ethanol (2.05 ± 0.21mgTEA/g of extract) and boiling water maceration (1.14 ± 0.01mgTEA/g of extract). In another study by Valadez-Carmona et al. (2018), the researchers reported that pressure and percentage of ethanol were the major factors that influenced the yield of phenolic compounds following the SFE of cocoa pod husk. The extract obtained at the optimum conditions (60 °C, 299 bar and 13.7% of ethanol) showed TPC of 12.97 mg GAE/g extract. Tyskiewicz et al. (2019) investigated the SC-CO_2 of phenolics from lavender flowers. The authors reported obtaining the highest TPC (10.17 mg GAE/g extract) at 60°C and a pressure of 250 bar after 45 min.

2.4.2.2 *Microemulsion extraction*

Microemulsion extraction is a sustainable and environmentally friendly technique with shorter process time than conventional extraction techniques. Other essential and distinctive features of microemulsion systems include but are not limited to droplet sizes from 1 to 100 nm, low viscosity, and optical transparency (Abbasi & Scanlon, 2016; Gadhave & Waghmare, 2014). The capacity of microemulsions to dissolve a large quantity of both hydrophilic and lipophilic compounds makes them a good choice for some vital food industry processes, such as extraction (Abbasi & Scanlon, 2016). Among several emulsifier-based extraction methods, microemulsion techniques (MET) represent a novel technique with potential application in extraction processes. Moreover, microemulsion techniques are capable of providing nanodroplets which act as receptors for various target compounds at a nanoscale level (Abbasi & Scanlon, 2016; Gadhave & Waghmare, 2014). The microemulsion technique uses an array of surfactants and has been employed to extract various bioactives and biomolecules including phenols, enzymes, and proteins (Materna & Szymanowski, 2002), oil (Abbasi & Radi, 2016; Teimouri et al., 2018), proteins, and glucosinolates from *Brassicaceae* oilseed meals (Ugolini et al., 2008). In the last few years, researchers have investigated the effectiveness of microemulsions to extract various organic and bioactive constituents. For example, canola seed oil extraction using a lecithin-based microemulsion system (Abbasi & Radi, 2016), β-carotene from carrot pomace using Tween 80 as a non-ionic surfactant (Roohinejad et al., 2014), and lutein from spinach leaves and marigold petals (Jalali Jivan & Abbasi, 2019). Therefore, there are opportunities for the application of this green approach in the extraction and recovery of bioactives from oilseeds co-products.

2.4.2.3 *Ultrasound-assisted extraction technique*

Ultrasound-assisted extraction (UAE) is one of the most popular extraction techniques, which utilizes acoustic cavitation leading to cell wall disruption and easier penetration of solvent, which in turn leads to the ultimate release of phytochemicals from the plant matrix. Some of the merits of UAE over conventional extraction methods include shorter extraction time, lesser use of solvents, automation, and better extraction efficiency when compared with conventional extraction methods (Chanioti & Tzia, 2017). In addition, UAE can be combined with green solvents, such as DES and ethanol, to extract phenolics and minor components from plant matrices (Chanioti & Tzia, 2018; Santana-Mayor et al., 2021). Ultrasound-aided extraction is advantageous over classical extraction methods in terms of overcoming inherent physical barriers, which are a hindrance to the complete extraction and isolation of endogenous phenolics. These physical barriers result from the interaction of phenolics with lignin, hulls, and cell walls, which are insoluble cellular constituents. For instance, sinapic acid occurs as glycosides, esters, and insoluble-bound forms, and this prevents the complete recovery from canola and mustard cakes. Ultrasound produces sound waves that create "cavitation bubbles" near the substrate, thereby resulting in cell wall disruption and the release of the bioactive constituents (Khoddami et al., 2013). A previous study by Teh and Birch (2014) concluded that the best conditions for the extraction of phenolics from de-oiled canola seed cakes were 200 W ultrasound extraction, solvent volume of 50 mL, 20 min extraction time and a temperature of 70°C. This method was found to be superior to conventional extraction methods because UAE has lower solvent consumption, cost, and improved antioxidant activity of the extracts. In a separate investigation by Szydłowska-Czerniak and Tulodzrecka (2014), the authors reported the optimum parameters for the extraction of phenolics and antioxidant compounds from rapeseed varieties using UAE were an extraction time of 13.8 min, a solvent-to-material ratio of 26.2 mL/g, and 50.3% solvent concentration. Dubie et al. (2013) conducted UAE of mustard meal phenolic antioxidants with the aid of a Branson Sonifier probe (input power of 400 W) using the following optimized conditions: temperature (75 °C), 20 min extraction time, solvent-to-meal ratio of 40:1, 70% ethanol, at 20 kHz and 0.5 W/mL ultrasound treatments. UAE has also been employed in the extraction of mustard's major sinapic acid and its derivatives. The technique manipulates the passage of ultrasonic waves into the sample-solvent mixture, creating cavitation bubbles which improve the extraction efficiency of phenolics. Szydłowska-Czerniak and Tulodzrecka (2015) used a UAE method to extract phenolic antioxidants from yellow mustard seed varieties, which resulted in the generation of considerable total phenolic content (27.16 mg/g SAE). UAE conditions of 40% ultrasound power, duration of 60 s and a single cycle with 70% (v/v) methanol were the optimum conditions for the maximum extraction and recovery of SADs from canola defatted meal after air frying pretreatment of the seeds (Fadairo et al., 2022).

2.4.2.4 Microwave-assisted extraction technique

Microwave-assisted extraction (MAE) as a green technique for the extraction of phenolic compounds plant materials gives rise to improved extraction efficiency when compared with classical solvent extraction. Nandasiri et al. (2023) studied the efficiency of MAE in the extraction of the main sinapic acid derivatives from defatted canola meal using 70%

(v/v) methanol and ethanol. The authors recorded a significant yield in canolol, an indication of the effectiveness of microwave extraction of phenolics from plant materials. Teh et al. (2015) studied microwave-assisted extraction of phenolic compounds from rapeseed cakes. The best conditions for the highest yield of phenolic compounds were 5 min duration, a solvent to sample proportion of 6 mL/g, and power of 633 W. The authors further concluded that this technique was rapid and economically viable. The successful application of MAE techniques in the extraction of bioactives from plant materials shows its efficacy and potential contributions as a green and novel technique.

2.4.2.5 *Pulsed-electric field extraction technique*

Pulsed-Electric Field (PEF) extraction is an emerging technology that uses high-voltage electric impulses, which result in the breakdown and permeability of the protoplasm to cellular components. The extraction efficiency of phenolics using PEF is influenced by factors including electric field intensity, amounts of pulses generated, and time. Teh et al. (2015) found the optimum extraction conditions for the highest recovery of phenolic derivatives from rapeseed cake as follows: exposure time of 10 min, voltage of 30 kV, and 30 Hz frequency. The authors also concluded that PEF extraction was superior to conventional methods because of its rapid extraction time and use of smaller volume of extraction solvent. A later investigation by Yu et al. (2016) used pulsed-electric field-aided extraction for the valorization of rapeseed leaves or green biomass. The authors revealed that the best conditions to obtain maximum total phenolic content (TPC) of pressed juices were pulse number of 200 and 8 kV/cm of pulse intensity.

2.4.2.6 *Deep eutectic solvents extraction*

The Deep Eutectic Solvent (DES) technique is a relatively new extraction method that has been gaining popularity as a viable and promising alternative to conventional organic solvent extraction (Cvjetko Bubalo et al., 2015). DES are hazardous-free solvents with outstanding properties such as little or no volatility at room temperature, miscibility with water, nonflammability, and high viscosity. They are effective solvents for the complete dissolution and extraction of a variety of nonpolar and polar compounds. A few studies have used DES for the extraction and separation of bioactive compounds of plant origin, including flavonoids (Bi et al., 2013; Dai et al., 2013; Nam et al., 2015), catechin (Heng & Kyungho, 2014), phenolic acids (Park et al., 2014), terpenoids, and saponin (Ribeiro et al., 2013). However, limited studies exist on the use of DES for the extraction of phenolic compounds from oilseeds. In addition, DES has also been combined with nonconventional extraction techniques such as microwave-assisted extraction (MAE) and ultrasound-assisted extraction (UAE) for extracting phenolic compounds. Besides their propensity to improve the extraction of phenolic compounds, assisted-extraction techniques using DES lower the overall volume of solvent used, decrease the operation costs, and shorten the extraction time. Đorđević et al. (2021) tested different DES solvents combinations, namely: triethanolamine: glycerol (TEOA: G), triethanolamine: propylene glycol (TEAO: PEG), and choline chloride: urea (ChCl: U) mixed with water and ethanol in a ratio of 1:4 v/v for the extraction of phenolic compounds from black mustard seeds. The authors recorded increased TPC and TFC which ranged from 19.9 ± 0.1 to 32.2 ± 0.2 mg GAE/g and 3.9 ± 0.1 to 7.4 ± 0.3 GAE/g, respectively. In the same study, the authors concluded that black mustard seed extracts obtained with the pure ChCl:U and the mixtures of ChCl:U or TEOA:G with ethanol exhibited the best antioxidant potential (IC50 = 100 mg/mL). The predominant antioxidant (canolol) in canola and mustard has been isolated and quantified using classical extraction methods. Based on the results of previous studies on other crops, there is potential in the adoption of DES as innovative and green solvents to improve the extraction and quantification of the phenolic compounds from mustard, canola seeds, and their by-products.

2.4.2.7 Enzyme-aided extraction

Enzyme-assisted extraction (EAE) has received increasing attention due to its environmental friendliness, healthy application, safety, and low cost in extraction of valuable compounds from plant materials (Grasso et al., 2012). The simultaneous production of high-quality oil and protein extracts constitute the most essential benefit of this technique. Moreover, the need for traditional degumming steps is eliminated in this process. Enzymatic treatment is also regarded as an effective way to improve hydrolysis and release bound molecules from the cellular matrices, thus leading to improved extraction, recovery, and ultimate reduction in solvent consumption. While there are various types of novel enzymes available in the industry for improving the extraction efficiency of oil and bioactive compounds from oilseeds, these enzymes need to be screened under controlled-environmental condition to ascertain their efficacy and functionality. The use of enzyme-assisted extraction as a rapid extraction and ecofriendly technique as an alternative to heat treatment in the biotransformation of phenolic derivatives, has been demonstrated (Morley et al., 2013).

Enzymic extractions produce specific products with high reproducibility. For example, horseradish peroxidase (HRP), an enzyme containing a porphyrin ring in which an iron atom is attached (Veitch, 2004), is located in the root of horseradish in the plant cell wall (Schloß et al., 1987). HRP is capable of oxidizing phenolic compounds (Kahn et al., 1995; Takahama & Oniki, 1994). It can also affect the oxidation of phenols with hydrogen peroxide to form phenoxy radicals. Such enzymes have been applied successfully for the hydrolysis of phenolic esters in cereals, for instance barley spent grain (Fujioka & Shibamoto, 2008). Khattab et al. (2014) reported a sequential extraction procedure for the production of canolol from canola through a sequence of alkaline/enzyme hydrolytic processes followed by decarboxylation of the hydrolyzed substrates under microwave irradiation. Cao et al. (2019) studied the in situ oxidation of sinapic acid from canola meal using tyrosinase and horseradish peroxidase (type II). The authors demonstrated the potential and suitability of these enzymes for the bioconversion of sinapic acid into oxidized compounds. EAE is regarded as an alternative method capable of catalyzing specific reactions and which is able to function optimally under moderate processing conditions (Shahid et al., 2016). A study by Odinot et al. (2017) used *Aspergillus niger* and *Neolentinus lepideus* to convert the sinapic acid to form canolol from the by-product matrix of the canola meal. The first step involved recombinant *Aspergillus niger* to produce feruloyl esterase type-A (AnFaeA) which released free sinapic acid from the meal by removing the esterified choline from sinapine and glucopyranosyl sinapate (Odinot et al., 2017). Once *Aspergillus niger* had liberated the free sinapic acid, the second step involved *Neolentinus lepideus*, which produced canolol from the liberated sinapic acid via a non-oxidative decarboxylation pathway. These authors reported that the conversation ratio from sinapic acid to canolol was above 80% (Odinot et al., 2017). An engineered sinapic acid decarboxylase was also used to produce canolol from sinapic acid (Morley et al., 2013).

2.4.2.8 Other extraction methods

The application of pressure contributes to the decarboxylation of sinapic acid to produce canolol (Li & Guo, 2016; Nandasiri et al., 2019; Nandasiri et al., 2021a, 2021b). Accelerated Solvent Extraction (ASE), also known as pressurized fluid extraction (PFE), is a novel technique that utilizes high pressure and moderate temperature to facilitate the extraction of phenolics from plant matrices. Moreover, the application of pressure also influences the breakdown of bonds in the cellular matrices, thus improving the recovery of phenolic compounds (Shahid et al., 2016). Nandasiri et al. (2019) employed ASE at high temperature (140–180°C) and pressure. The authors reported an improved extraction yields of phenolics as well as the antioxidant activity of the extracts.

2.5 Summary and conclusion

Canolol and its derivatives have garnered considerable attention in recent times due to their high-antioxidant and health-promoting properties. But more research needs to be conducted in this specific area to better understand the efficacy of this phenolic compound on human health. Our initial studies found that canolol has specific extractability requirements using different processing conditions on different oilseed varieties. Moreover, its derivatives, including dimers and trimers, have yet to be fully investigated for both antioxidant and other health-promoting factors. Their high reactivity and oxidation ability may limit their use in the food and nutraceutical industries. However, with the application of esterification and creating a better delivery system, canolol could be incorporated into the food systems as a natural antioxidant for preventing lipid oxidation. Future development for a suitable delivery system for these antioxidants is needed so they can be introduced into the body to mitigate many physiological conditions including cancers. Consequently, with the development of advanced technology and combined processing techniques, canolol can play an important role in both the food and nutraceutical industries.

References

Aachary, A. A., Chen, Y., Eskin, N. A. M., Thiyam-Hollander, U. (2014). Crude canolol and canola distillate extracts improve the stability of refined canola oil during deep-fat frying. *European Journal of Lipid Science and Technology, 116* (11), 1467–1476. https://doi.org/10.1002/ejlt.201300498

Abbasi, S., Radi, M. (2016). Food grade microemulsion systems: Canola oil/lecithin: n-propanol/water. *Food Chemistry, 194,* 972–979. https://doi.org/10.1016/J.FOODCHEM.2015.08.078

Abbasi, S., Scanlon, M. G. (2016). Nanostructural characterization of food grade microemulsions: ultrasonic resonator technology. *Emulsions,* 443–478. https://doi.org/10.1016/B978-0-12-804306-6.00013-1

Belwal, T., Ezzat, S. M., Rastrelli, L., Bhatt, I. D., Daglia, M., Baldi, A., Devkota, H. P., Orhan, I. E., Patra, J. K., Das, G., Anandharamakrishnan, C., Gomez-Gomez, L., Nabavi, S. F., Nabavi, S. M., Atanasov, A. G. (2018). A critical analysis of extraction techniques used for botanicals: Trends, priorities, industrial uses, and optimization strategies. In *TrAC - Trends in Analytical Chemistry* (Vol. 100, pp. 82–102). Elsevier B.V. https://doi.org/10.1016/j.trac.2017.12.018

Bi, W., Tian, M., Row, K. H. (2013). Evaluation of alcohol-based deep eutectic solvent in extraction and determination of flavonoids with response surface methodology optimization. *Journal of Chromatography A, 1285,* 22–30. https://doi.org/10.1016/j.chroma.2013.02.041

Bubalo, M. C., Vidoviic, S., Radojcic, I. R., Jokic, S. (2015). Green solvents for green technologies. *Journal of Chemical Technology and Biotechnology. 90*(9), 1631–1639. https://doi.org/10.1002/jctb.4668

Cao, X., Liang, J., Aluko, R. E., Thiyam-Holländer, U. (2019). In situ oxidation of canola meal sinapic acid by horseradish peroxidase (type II) and tyrosinase. *Journal of Food Biochemistry, 43*(6), e12884. https://doi.org/10.1111/JFBC.12884

Cao, X., Tsiokamoto, T., Seki, T., Tanaka, H., Morimura, S., Cao, L., Mizoshita, T., Ban, H., Toyoda, T., Maeda, H., Tatematsu, M. (2008). 4-Vinyl-2,6-dimethoxyphenol (canolol) suppresses oxidative stress and gastric carcinogenesis in *Helicobacter pylori*-infested carcinogen-treated Mongolian gerbils. *International Journal of Cancer, 122*(7), 1445–1454. https://doi.org/10.1002/ijc.23245

Castro-Vargas, H. I., Baumann, W., Ferreira, S. R. S., Parada-Alfonso, F. (2019). Valorization of papaya (Carica papaya L.) agroindustrial waste through the recovery of phenolic antioxidants by supercritical fluid extraction. *Journal of Food Science and Technology, 56*(6), 3055–3066.

Chadni, M., Flourat, A. L., Reungoat, V., Mouterde, L. M. M., Allais, F., Ioannou, I. (2021). Selective extraction of sinapic acid derivatives from mustard seed meal by acting on pH: Toward a high antioxidant activity rich extract. *Molecules, 26*(1)

Chanioti, S., Tzia, C. (2017). Optimization of ultrasound-assisted extraction of oil from olive pomace using response surface technology: Oil recovery, unsaponifiable matter, total phenol content and antioxidant activity. *LWT - Food Science and Technology, 79*, 178–189. https://doi.org/10.1016/J.LWT.2017.01.029

Chanioti, S., Tzia, C. (2018). Extraction of phenolic compounds from olive pomace by using natural deep eutectic solvents and innovative extraction techniques. *Innovative Food Science & Emerging Technologies, 48*, 228–239. https://doi.org/10.1016/J.IFSET.2018.07.001

Chemat, F. O., Vorobiev, E. Q. (2019). *Food Processing Techniques. Preservation, Transformation nd Extraction*. Academic Press.

Cvjetko Bubalo, M., Vidović, S., Radojčić Redovniković, I., Jokić, S. (2015). Green solvents for green technologies. *Journal of Chemical Technology and Biotechnology, 90*(9), 1631–1639. https://doi.org/10.1002/jctb.4668

Dai, Y., Van Spronsen, J., Witkamp, G.-J., Verpoorte, R., Choi, Y. H. (2013). Natural deep eutectic solvents as new potential media for green technology. *Analytica Chimica Acta, 766*, 61–68. https://doi.org/10.1016/j.aca.2012.12.019

De Melo, M. M. R., Silvestre, A. J. D., Silva, C. M. (2014). Supercritical fluid extraction of vegetable matrices: Applications, trends, and future perspectives of a convincing green technology. *The Journal of Supercritical Fluids, 92*, 115–176. https://doi.org/10.1016/J.SUPFLU.2014.04.007

Đorđević, B. S., Todorović, Z. B., Troter, D. Z., Stanojević, L. P., Stojanović, G. S., Đalović, I. G., Mitrović, P. M., Veljković, V. B. (2021). Extraction of phenolic compounds from black mustard (*Brassica nigra* L.) seed by deep eutectic solvents. *Journal of Food Measurement and Characterization, 15*(2), 1931–1938.

Dubie, J., Stancik, A., Morra, M., Nindo, C. (2013). Antioxidant extraction from mustard (brassica juncea) seed meal using high-intensity ultrasound. *Journal of Food Science, 78*(4), 542–548. https://doi.org/10.1111/1750-3841.12085

Dunford, N. T. (2012). Food and industrial bioproducts and bioprocessing. In *Food and Industrial Bioproducts and Bioprocessing*. https://doi.org/10.1002/9781119946083

Engels, C., Schieber, A., Gänzle, M. G. (2012). Sinapic acid derivatives in defatted Oriental mustard (*Brassica juncea* L.) seed meal extracts using UHPLC-DAD-ESI-MS n and identification of compounds with antibacterial activity. *European Food Research and Technology, 234*(3), 535–542. https://doi.org/10.1007/S00217-012-1669-Z

Eskin, N. A. M. (2020). Canada's Cinderella crop. *Food Science and Technology, 34*(2), 49–51. https://doi.org/10.1002/fsat.3402_13.x

Essien, S. O., Young, B., Baroutian, S. (2020). Recent advances in subcritical water and supercritical carbon dioxide extraction of bioactive compounds from plant materials. *Trends in Food Science & Technology, 97*, 156–169. https://doi.org/10.1016/J.TIFS.2020.01.014

Fadairo, O., Nandasiri, R., Alashi, A. M., Eskin, N. A. M., Thiyam-Holländer, U. (2021). Air frying pretreatment and the recovery of lipophilic sinapates from the oil fraction of mustard samples. *Journal of Food Science, 86*, 3810–3823. https://doi.org/10.1111/1750-3841.15861

Fadairo, O. S., Nandasiri, R., Eskin, N. A. M., Aluko, R. E., Scanlon, M. G. (2023). Air frying as a heat treatment method for improving the extraction and yield of canolol from canola seed oil. *Food and Bioprocess Technology, 16*(3), 639–651. https://doi.org/10.1007/s11947-022-02961-7

Fadairo, O. S., Nandasiri, R., Nguyen, T., Eskin, N. A. M., Aluko, R. E., Scanlon, M. G. (2022). Improved extraction efficiency and antioxidant activity of defatted canola meal extract phenolic compounds obtained from air-fried seeds. *Antioxidants, 11*, 2411. https://doi.org/10.3390/ANTIOX11122411

Fang, J., Seki, T., Tsukamoto, T., Quin, H., Yin, H., Liao, L., Nakamura, H., Maeda, H. (2013). Protection from inflammatory bowel disease andcolitis0associated carcinogenesis with 4-vinyl 2,6-dimethoxyphenol (canolol) involves suppression of oxidative stress and inflammatory cytokine. *Carcinogenesis, 34*(12), 2833–2841. https://doi.org/10.1093/carcin/bgt309

Ferrentino, G., Morozova, K., Mosibo, O. K., Ramezani, M., Scampicchio, M. (2018). Biorecovery of antioxidants from apple pomace by supercritical fluid extraction. *Journal of Cleaner Production, 186*, 253–261. https://doi.org/10.1016/j.jclepro.2018.03.165

Fujioka, K., Shibamoto, T. (2008). Chlorogenic acid and caffeine contents in various commercial brewed coffees. *Food Chemistry, 106*(1), 217–221.

Gadhave, A. D., Waghmare, J. T. (2014). A short review on microemulsion and its application in extraction of vegetable oil. *IJRET: International Journal of Research in Engineering and Technology*. http://www.ijret.org

Galano, A., Francisco-Ma′rquez, M., Ivarez-Idaboy, J. R. (2011). Canolol: A promising chemical agent against oxidative stress. *Journal of Physical Chemistry B, 115*, 8590–8596.

Grasso, F. V., Montoya, P. A., Camusso, C. C., Maroto, B. G. (2012). Improvement of soybean oil solvent extraction through enzymatic pretreatment. *International Journal of Agronomy, 2012*, 1–7. https://doi.org/10.1155/2012/543230

Harbaum-Piayda, B., Oehlke, K., Sönnichsen, F. D., Zacchi, P., Eggers, R., Schwarz, K. (2010). New polyphenolic compounds in commercial deodistillate and rapeseed oils. *Food Chemistry, 123*(3), 607–615. https://doi.org/10.1016/J.FOODCHEM.2010.04.078

Heng, Z., Kyungho, R. (2014). Extraction of catechin compounds from green tea with a new green solvent. *Chem. Res. Chin. Univ, 30*(1), 37–41. https://doi.org/10.1007/s40242-014-3339-0

Hudson, E. A., Dinh, P. A., Kokubun, T., Simmonds, M. S., Gescher, A. (2000). Higher radical scavenging activities of polyphenolic antioxidants can be ascribed to chemical reaction following their oxidation. *Biochimica et Biophysica Acta, 1572*(1), 123–132. https://doi.org/10.1016/S0304-4165(02)00285-4

Ishtiaque, S., Khan, N., Siddiqui, M. A., Siddiqi, R., Naz, S. (2013). Antioxidant potential of the extracts, fractions and oils derived from oilseeds. *Antioxidants, 2*, 246–256. https://doi.org/10.3390/antiox2040246

Jalali Jivan, M., Abbasi, S. (2019). An attempt to cast light into lutein extraction and its alkali optimization. *Journal of Food Measurement and Characterization, 13*(1), 154–161.

Jenab, E., Temelli, F., Curtis, J. M. (2013). Lipase-catalysed interesterification between canola oil and fully hydrogenated canola oil in contact with supercritical carbon dioxide. *Food Chemistry, 141*(3), 2220–2228. https://doi.org/10.1016/J.FOODCHEM.2013.04.079

Kahn, V., Lindner, P., Zakin, V. (1995). Kojic acid conversion to a yellow product(s) via the horseradish peroxidase/H_2O_2 system1. *Journal of Food Biochemistry, 19*(1), 67–80. https://doi.org/10.1111/J.1745-4514.1995.TB00521.X

Kampa, M., Alexaki, V-I., Notas, G., Nifli, A-P., Nistikaki, A., Hatzoglou, A., Bakogeorgou, E., Kouimtzoglou, E., Biekas, C., Boskou, D., Gravanis, A., Castanon, E. 2003. Antiproliferative and apoptotic effects of selective phenolic acids on T47D human breast cells: Potential mechanisms of action. *Breast Cancer Research, 6*(2), 1–12.

Keyhani, A., Yaylayan, V. A. (2002). Glycine specific novel maillard reaction products: 5-hydroxy-1,3-dimethyl-2(1 H)-quinoxalinone and related compounds. *Journal of Agricultural and Food Chemistry, 45*(3), 697–702. https://doi.org/10.1021/jf960528g

Khattab, R., Michael, Eskin, Thiyam-Hollander, U. (2014). Production of canolol from canola meal phenolics via hydrolysis and microwave-induced decarboxylation. *JAOCS, Journal of the American Oil Chemists' Society, 91*, 89–97. https://doi.org/10.1007/s11746-013-2345-6

Khattab, R. Y., Eskin, M. N. A., Thiyam-Hollander, U. (2013). Production of canolol from canola meal phenolics via hydrolysis and microwave-induced decarboxylation. *Journal of the American Oil Chemists' Society, 91*(1), 89–97. https://doi.org/10.1007/S11746-013-2345-6

Khoddami, A., Wilkes, M. A., Roberts, T. H. (2013). Techniques for analysis of plant phenolic compounds. In *Molecules* (Vol. 18, Issue 2, pp. 2328–2375). https://doi.org/10.3390/molecules18022328

Koski, A., Pekkarinen, S., Hopia, A., Wahala, K., Heinonen, M. (2003). Processing of rapeseed oil: Effects on sinapic acid derivative content and oxidative stability. *European Journal of Lipid Science and Technology, 217*(2), 110–114.

Kozlowska, H., Naczk, M., Shahidi, F., Zadernowski, R. (1990). Phenolic acids and tannins in rapeseed and canola. *Canola and Rapeseed*, 193–210. https://doi.org/10.1007/978-1-4615-3912-4_11

Kozlowska, M., Gruczynska, E., Scibisz, I. S., Rudzinska, M. (2016). Fatty acids and sterols composition, and antioxidant activity of oils extracted from plant seeds. *Food Chemistry, 213*, 450–456.

Kraljić, K., Brkan, V., Škevin, D., Srček, V. G., Radošević, K. (2019). Canolol dimer, a biologically active phenolic compound of edible rapeseed oil. *Lipids, 54*(2–3), 189–200. https://doi.org/10.1002/lipd.12132

Kraljić, K., Škevin, D., Barišić, L., Kovačević, M., Obranović, M., Jurčević, I. (2015). Changes in 4-vinylsyringol and other phenolics during rapeseed oil refining. *Food Chemistry, 187*, 236–242. https://doi.org/10.1016/j.foodchem.2015.04.039

Kumar, S. P. J., Prasad, S. R., Banerjee, R., Agarwal, D. K., Kulkarni, K. S., Ramesh, K. V. (2017). Green solvents and technologies for oil extraction from oilseeds. *Chemistry Central Journal, 11*(1), 1–7. https://doi.org/10.1186/s13065-017-0238-8

Kuwahara, H., Kanazawa, A., Wakamatu, D., Morimura, S., Kida, K., Akaike, T., Maeda, H. (2004). *Antioxidative and antimutagenic activities of 4-Vinyl-2,6-dimethoxyphenol (canolol) isolated from canola oil*. https://doi.org/10.1021/jf040045

Lawrence, T. (2009). The nuclear factor NJ-Kappa B pathway in inflammation. *Cold Spring Harbor Perspectives in Biology, 1*(6). https://doi.org/10.1101/cshperspect.a001651

Li, J., Guo, Z. (2016). Identification and quantification of phenolic compounds in rapeseed originated lecithin and antioxidant activity evaluation. *LWT - Food Science and Technology, 73*, 397–405. https://doi.org/10.1016/j.lwt.2016.06.039

Liu, T., Zhang, L., Joo, D., Sun, S. C. (2017). NF-κB signaling in inflammation. *Signal Transduction and Targeted Therapy*, *2*(1), 1–9. https//doi.org/1038/sigtrans.2017.23

Lohani, U., Fallahi, P., Muthukumarappan (2015). comparison of ethyl acetate with hexane for oil extraction from various oilseeds. *Journal of the American Oil Chemist's Society*, *92*(5), 743–754.

Materna, K., Szymanowski, J. (2002). Separation of phenols from aqueous micellar solutions by cloud point extraction. *Journal of Colloid and Interface Science*, *255*(1), 195–201. https://doi.org/10.1006/JCIS.2002.8613

Matthäus, B., Pudel, F., Chen, Y., Achary, A., Thiyam-Holländer, U. (2014). Impact of canolol-enriched extract from heat-treated canola meal to enhance oil quality parameters in deep-frying: A comparison with rosemary extract and TBHQ-fortified oil systems. *Journal of the American Oil Chemists' Society*, *91*(12), 2065–2076. https://doi.org/10.1007/s11746-014-2561-8

Mayengbam, S., Aachary, A., Thiyam-Hollander, U. (2014). Endogenous phenolics in hulls and cotyledons of mustard and canola: A comparative study on its sinapates and antioxidant capacity. *Antioxidants*, *3*(3), 544–558. https://doi.org/10.3390/antiox3030544

Morley, K. L., Grosse, S., Leisch, H., Lau, P. C. K. (2013). Antioxidant canolol production from a renewable feedstock via an engineered decarboxylase. *Green Chemistry*, *15*(12), 3312–3317. https://doi.org/10.1039/C3GC40748A

Mukhopadhyay, M. (2000). *Natural extracts using supercritical carbon dioxide*. CRC Press. https://doi.org/10.1201/9781420041699

Murtaza, G., Latifi, U., Najam-Ui-Haq, M., Sajjad, A., Karim, S., Akhtar, M., Hussain, I. (2013). Resveratrol: An active compounds in red wines for health. *Journal of Food and Drug Analysis*, *21*(1). https://doi.org/10.6227/jfda.2013210101

Nam, M. W., Zhao, J., Lee, M. S., Jeong, J. H., Lee, J. (2015). Enhanced extraction of bioactive natural products using tailor-made deep eutectic solvents: Application to flavonoid extraction from *Flos sophorae*. *Green Chemistry*, *17*(3), 1718–1727. https://doi.org/10.1039/c4gc01556h

Nandasiri, R., Eskin, N. A. M. (2022). Canolol and its derivatives: A novel bioactive with antioxidant and anticancer properties. *Advances in Food and Nutrition Research*, *100*, 109–129. https://doi.org/10.1016/BS.AFNR.2022.03.003

Nandasiri, R., Eskin, N. A. M., Komatsu, E., Perreault, H., Thiyam-Holländer, U. (2021a). Valorization of canola by-products: Concomitance of flavor-active bitter phenolics using pressurized heat treatments. *LWT*, *138*, 110397. https://doi.org/10.1016/J.LWT.2020.110397

Nandasiri, R., Eskin, N. A. M., Thiyam-Höllander, U. (2019). Antioxidative polyphenols of canola meal extracted by high pressure: Impact of temperature and solvents. *Journal of Food Science*, *84*(11), 3117–3128. https://doi.org/10.1111/1750-3841.14799

Nandasiri, R., Fadairo, O., Nguyen, T., Zago, E., Anas, M. U. M., Eskin, N. A. M. (2023). Optimization of canolol production from canola meal using microwave digestion as a pre-treatment method. *Foods*, *12*(2), 318. https://doi.org/10.3390/foods12020318

Nandasiri, R., Imran, A., Thiyam-Holländer, U., Eskin, N. A. M. (2021b). Rapidoxy® 100: A solvent-free pre-treatment for production of canolol. *Frontiers in Nutrition*, 399. https://doi.org/10.3389/FNUT.2021.687851

Nandasiri, R., Zago, E., Thiyam-Holländer, U., Eskin, N. A. M. (2021c). Attenuation of sinapic acid and sinapine-derived flavor-active compounds using a factorial-based pressurized high-temperature processing. *Journal of the American Oil Chemists' Society*, *98*(7), 779–794. https: / / doi.org/10.1002/AOCS.12510

Nautiyal, O. H. (2016). *Cronicon Open Access Chemistry*. Review Article Food Processing by supercritical carbon dioxide-Review.

Nguyen, T., Nandasiri, R., Fadairo, O., Eskin, M. N. A. (2023). The effect of pH on the phenolic content and antioxidant properties of three different mustard extracts. *Journal of Food Science, 88*(7), 2882–2901. https://doi.org/10.1111/1750-3841.16655

Odinot, E., Fine, F., Sigoillot, J. C., Navarro, D., Laguna, O., Bisotto, A., Peyronnet, C., Ginies, C., Lecomte, J., Faulds, C. B., Lomascolo, A. (2017). A two-step bioconversion process for canolol production from rapeseed meal combining an *Aspergillus niger* feruloyl esterase and the fungus *Neolentinus lepideus. Microorganisms, 5*(4), 1–17. https://doi.org/10.3390/microorganisms5040067

Park, H. E., Tang, B., Row, K. H. (2014). Application of deep eutectic solvents as additives in ultrasonic extraction of two phenolic acids from herba *Artemisiae Scopariae. Analytical Letters, 47*(9), 1476–1484. https://doi.org/10.1080/00032719.2013.874016

Rasera, G. B., Hilkner, M. H., Alencar, S. M., Janser, R. (2019). Biologically active compounds from white and black mustard grains. An optimization study for recovery and identification of phenolic antioxidants. *Industrial Crops and Products, 135*, 294–300. https://doi.org/10.1016/j.indcrop.2019.04.059

Ribeiro, B. D., Coelho, M. A. Z., Marrucho, I. M. (2013). Extraction of saponins from sisal (*Agave sisalana*) and juá (*Ziziphus joazeiro*) with cholinium-based ionic liquids and deep eutectic solvents. *European Food Research and Technology, 237*(6), 965–975.

Roohinejad, S., Oey, I., Everett, D. W., Niven, B. E. (2014). evaluating the effectiveness of β-carotene extraction from pulsed electric field-treated carrot pomace using oil-in-water microemulsion. *Food and Bioprocess Technology, 7*(11), 3336–3348.

Santana-Mayor, Á., Rodríguez-Ramos, R., Herrera-Herrera, A. V., Socas-Rodríguez, B., Rodríguez-Delgado, M. Á. (2021). Deep eutectic solvents. The new generation of green solvents in analytical chemistry. *TrAC Trends in Analytical Chemistry, 134*, 116108. https://doi.org/10.1016/J.TRAC.2020.116108

Sato, T., Ikeya, Y., Adachi, S. I., Yagasaki, K., Nihei, K. I., Itoh, N. (2019). Extraction of strawberry leaves with supercritical carbon dioxide and entrainers: Antioxidant capacity, total phenolic content, and inhibitory effect on uric acid production of the extract. *Food and Bioproducts Processing, 117*, 160–169

Schloß, P., Walter, C., Mäder, M. (1987). Basic peroxidases in isolated vacuoles of nicotiana tabacum L. *Planta, 170*(2), 225–229.

Shahid, M., Yusuf, M., Mohammad, F. (2016). Plant phenolics: A review on modern extraction techniques. *Recent Progress in Medicinal Plants, 41*(11), 265–287. https://www.researchgate.net/publication/310614780

Shrestha, K., Stevens, C. V., De Meulenaer, B. (2012). Isolation and Identification of a Potent Radical Scavenger (Canolol) from Roasted High Erucic Mustard Seed Oil from Nepal and Its Formation during Roasting. *Journal of Agricultural and Food Chemistry, 60*(30), 7506–7512. https://doi.org/10.1021/jf301738y

Shuklah, Y., Singh, R. (2011). Resveratrol and cellular mechanisms of cancer prevention. *Annals of the New York Academy of Sciences, 1215*(1), 1–8. https://doi.org/10.1111/j.1749-6632.2010.05870.x

Siger, A., Gawrysiak-Witulska, M, Bartkowiak-Broda, I. (2017). Antioxidant (tocopherol and canolol) content in rapeseed oil obtained from roasted yellow-seeded Brassica napus. *Journal of the American Oil Chemist's Society, 94*(1), 3246, https://doi.org/10.1007/s11746-016-2921-7

Spielmeyer, A., Wagner, A., Jahreis, G. (2009). Influence of thermal treatment of rapeseed on the canolol content. *Food Chemistry, 112*(4), 944–948. https://doi.org/10.1016/j.foodchem.2008.07.011

Sun, M., Xu, L., Saldana, M.D.A., Temelli, F. (2008). Comparison of canola meals obtained with conventional methods and supercritical CO2 with and without ethanol. *Journal of the American Oil Chemist's Society, 85*, 667–675.

Szydłowska-Czerniak, A., Tulodzrecka, A. (2014). Antioxidant capacity of rapeseed extracts obtained by conventional and ultrasound-assisted extraction. *Journal of the American Oil Chemist's Society, 91*(12), 2011–2019, https://doi.org/10.1007/S11746-014-2557-4

Szydłowska-Czerniak, A., Tulodzrecka, A. (2015). Application of response surface methodology to optimize ultrasound-assisted extraction of total antioxidants from *Brassica napus* cultivars. *European Journal of Lipid Science and Technology, 117*(4), 491–502. https://doi.org/10.1002/ejlt.201400310

Takahama, U., Oniki, T. (1994). Effects of ascorbate on the oxidation of derivatives of hydroxycinnamic acid and the mechanism of oxidation of sinapic acid by cell wall-bound peroxidases. *Plant and Cell Physiology, 35*(4), 593–600. https://doi.org/10.1093/OXFORDJOURNALS.PCP.A078634

Teh, S. S., Birch, E. J. (2014). Effect of ultrasonic treatment on the polyphenol content and antioxidant capacity of extract from defatted hemp, flax, and canola seed cakes. *Ultrasonics Sonochemistry, 21*(1), 346–353. https://doi.org/10.1016/J.ULTSONCH.2013.08.002

Teh, S. S., Niven, B. E., Bekhit, A. E. D. A., Carne, A., Birch, E. J. (2015). Microwave and pulsed electric field assisted extractions of polyphenols from defatted canola seed cake. *International Journal of Food Science Technology, 50*(5), 1109–1115. https://doi.org/10.1111/IJFS.12749

Teimouri, S., Abbasi, S., Scanlon, M. G. (2018). Stabilisation mechanism of various inulins and hydrocolloids: Milk–sour cherry juice mixture. *International Journal of Dairy Technology, 71*(1), 208–215. https://doi.org/10.1111/1471-0307.12376

Texeira, J., Gaspar, A., Garrido, E.M., Garrido, J., Borges, F. (2013). Hydroxycinnamic acid antioxidants. An electrochemical overview. *Biomed Research International*, 2013. https://doi.org/10.1155/2013/251754

Thiyam, U., Claudia, P., Jan, U., Alfred, B. (2009). De-oiled rapeseed and a protein isolate: characterization of sinapic acid derivatives by HPLC–DAD and LC–MS. *European Food Research and Technology, 229*(5), 825–831. https://doi.org/10.1007/s00217-009-1122-0

Thiyam, U., Kuhlmann, A., Stöckmann, H., Schwarz, K. (2004). Prospects of rapeseed oil by-products with respect to antioxidative potential. *Comptes Rendus Chimie, 7*(6–7), 611–616. https://doi.org/10.1016/J.CRCI.2004.02.011

Thiyam, U., Stockmann, H., Felde, T. Z., Schwartz, K. (2006). Antioxidative effect of the main sinapic acid derivatives from rapeseed and mustard oil by-products. *European Journal of Lipid Science and Technology, 108*(3), 239–248. https://doi.org/10.1002/EJLT.200500292

Thiyam-Holländer, U., Aladedunye, F., Logan, A., Yang, H., Diehl, B. W. K. (2014). Identification and quantification of canolol and related sinapate precursors in Indian mustard oils and Canadian mustard products. *European Journal of Lipid Science and Technology, 116*(12), 1664–1674. https://doi.org/10.1002/EJLT.201400222

Tuhanioglu, A., Ubeyitogullari, A. (2022). Extraction of high-value lipids and phenolic compounds from sorghum bran via a sequential supercritical carbon dioxide approach. *ACS Food Science and Technology.* https://doi.org/10.1021/acsfoodscitech.2c00266

Tyskiewicz, K., Konkol, M., Rój, E. (2019). Supercritical carbon dioxide (SC-CO2) extraction of phenolic compounds from lavender *(Lavandula angustifolia)* flowers: A box-behnken experimental optimization. *Molecules, 24*(18). https://doi.org/10.3390/molecules24183354

Ugolini, L., De Nicola, G., Palmieri, S. (2008). Use of reverse micelles for the simultaneous extraction of oil, proteins, and glucosinolates from cruciferous oilseeds. *Journal of Agricultural and Food Chemistry, 56*(5), 1595–1601. https://doi.org/10.1021/JF072582A

Valadez-Carmona, L., Ortiz-Moreno, A., Ceballos-Reyes, G., Mendiola, J. A., Ibáñez, E. (2018). Valorization of cacao pod husk through supercritical fluid extraction of phenolic compounds. *The Journal of Supercritical Fluids, 131*, 99–105. https://doi.org/10.1016/J.SUPFLU.2017.09.011

Veitch, N. C. (2004). Horseradish peroxidase: a modern view of a classic enzyme. *Phytochemistry, 65*(3), 249–259. https://doi.org/10.1016/J.PHYTOCHEM.2003.10.022

Wakamatsu, D., Morimura, S., Sawa, T., Kida, K., Nakai, C., Maeda, H. (2005). Isolation, identification, and structure of a potent alkyl-peroxyl radical scavenger in crude canola oil, canolol. *Bioscience, Biotechnology, and Biochemistry, 69*(8), 1568–1574. https://doi.org/10.1271/bbb.69.1568

Wang, W., Rao, L., Wu, X., Wang, Y., Zhao, L., Liao, X. (2021). Supercritical carbon dioxide applications in food processing. In *Food Engineering Reviews* (Vol. 13, Issue 3, pp. 570–591). Springer. https://doi.org/10.1007/s12393-020-09270-9

Wijesundera, C., Ceccato, C., Fagan, P., Shen, Z. (2008). Seed roasting improves the oxidative stability of canola (*B. napus*) and mustard (*B. juncea*) seed oils. *European Journal of Lipid Science and Technology, 110*(4), 3690. https://doi.org/10.1002/ejlt.200700214

Yang, M., Zheng, C., Zhou, Q., Liu, C., Li, W., Huang, F. (2014). Influence of microwaves treatment of rapeseed on phenolic compounds and canolol content. *Journal of Agricultural and Food Chemistry, 62*(8), 1956–1963. https://doi.org/10.1021/jf4054287

Yu, X., Gouyo, T., Grimi, N., Bals, O., Vorobiev, E. (2016). Pulsed electric field pretreatment of rapeseed green biomass (stems) to enhance pressing and extractives recovery. *Bioresource Technology, 199*, 194–201. https://doi.org/10.1016/J.BIORTECH.2015.08.073

Zhang, H., Sun, S. C. (2015). NF-κB in inflammation and renal diseases. *Cell and Bioscience. 5*(1), 1–12.

Zhang, X., Heinonen, S., Levanen, E. (2014). Applications of supercritical carbon dioxide in materials processing and synthesis. *RSC Advances, 4*(105), 61137–61152.

chapter three

Analysis of canolol (4-vinylsyringol) and its derivatives in rapeseed oil and sidestreams

Karin Schwarz

3.1 Introduction

The occurrence of canolol (4-vinyl-2,6-dimethoxyphenol, 4-vinylsyringol) was observed in the early 2000s by Koski et al. (2003) and Wakamatsu et al. (2005) without it being immediately clear the relationship between 4-vinylsyringol formation and sinapic acid content in rapeseed (Figure 3.1).

Today, it has been documented in many studies that 4-vinylsyringol arises from sinapic acid, which in turn belongs to the hydroxycinnamic acid group and, with its derivatives, is the most important phenolic compound in rapeseed. The content of sinapic acid derivatives is about 8–20 g/kg of rapeseed and canola. Other cinnamic acids present in small amounts in rapeseed are ferula, coumaric, vanillic, syringic, and 3- and 2-hydroxybenzoic acids.

In rapeseed, the occurrence of sinapic acid is reported as free acid (6%–14%), bound to glucose as well as choline ester (70%–90%); the latter is called sinapine. Furthermore, sinapic acid occurs in various glycosidic conjugates and as malate in smaller amounts (Siger et al. 2008; Liu et al. 2012)

During the processing of rapeseed into rapeseed oil and its sidestream products, there is a release of sinapine from its derivatives and a degradation of sinapic acid. Decarboxylation results in the formation of 4-vinylsyringol. Chemical synthesis by decarboxylation was described by Fiddler et al. (1967) and Bernini et al. (2007). Vinylsyringol is of interest to the food industry due to its flavors and antioxidant effects (Oehlke et al. 2017). In addition, numerous biological effects of vinylsyringol have been reported, including antimutagenic, anti-inflammatory, and anticarcinogenic activity (Kuwahara et al. 2004; Kraljić et al. 2019).

Further, 4-vinylsyringol is of interest as a starting substance for epoxy compounds in the field of coatings and overlays in the technical sector. Diepoxidized diphenyls from vinylsyringol are able to replace bisphenol

DOI: 10.1201/b22828-3

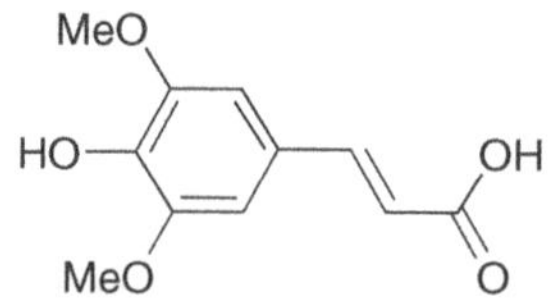

sinapic acid (1)

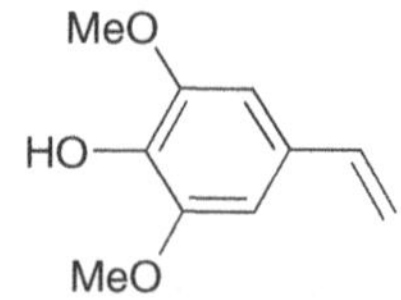

4-vinylsyringol (2)

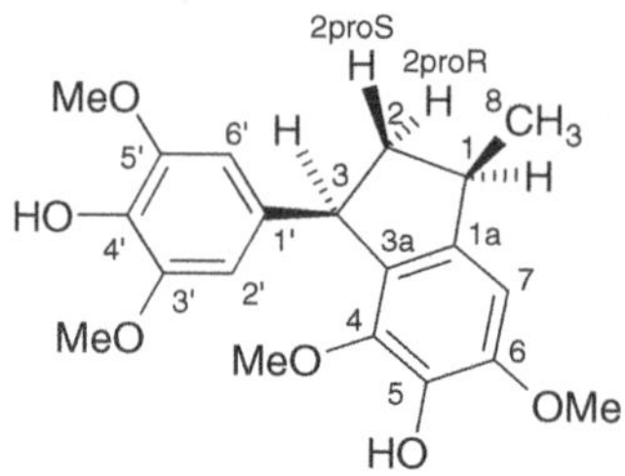

cis-diastereomer of phenylindane (3a)

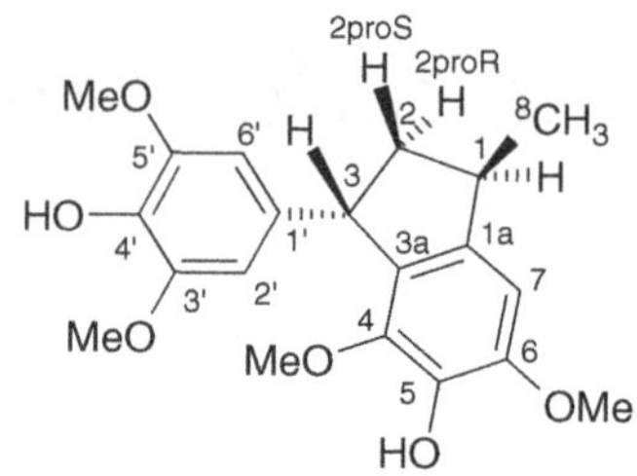

trans-diastereomer of phenylindane (3a)

Figure 3.1 Sinapic acid (1), 4-vinylsyringol (2) and 4-vinylsyringol dimer (3a cis- and 3b trans-diastereomers of phenylindane). (Harbaum-Piayda et al. 2010).

A and at the same time have a much lower hormonal potential; tested was the affinity to the estrogen receptor ERα by molecular docking calculation (Zago et al. 2016).

4-Vinylsyringol is formed in particular under the influence of elevated temperatures during the processing of rapeseed into rapeseed oil. Since 4-vinylsyringol is very reactive, it can react further with other substances to form new compounds. Among others, Rein et al. (2005) described the intercation of 4-vinylsyringol and anthocyanins. 4-Vinylsyringol can dimerize under the influence of elevated temperatures, so that relevant contents occur in oil and side products. Trimers, on the other hand, are only formed in very small quantities and their occurrence has only been described by a few authors to date (Harbaum-Piayda et al. 2010).

Dimerization often occurs for simple phenolic compounds such as hydroxycinnamic acids in nature by binding to plant cell walls. Binding can occur either via radical coupling mechanism or via a photochemical reaction. Under heat, formation could follow a process described by Frank et al. (2007) for the dimerization of vinylcatechol by forming an oxionium ion as an intermediate. Aldabalde et al. (2011) suggested that the formation proceeds in an acid-catalyzed manner. In this process, 4-vinylsyringol is protonated to form a stable carbocation, which in turn undergoes cationic dimerization with a second molecule of 4-vinylsyringol (Figure 3.2). Subsequently, intramolecular ring closure occurs via electrophilic aromatic substitution, resulting in an indane structure (Kraljić et al. 2015).

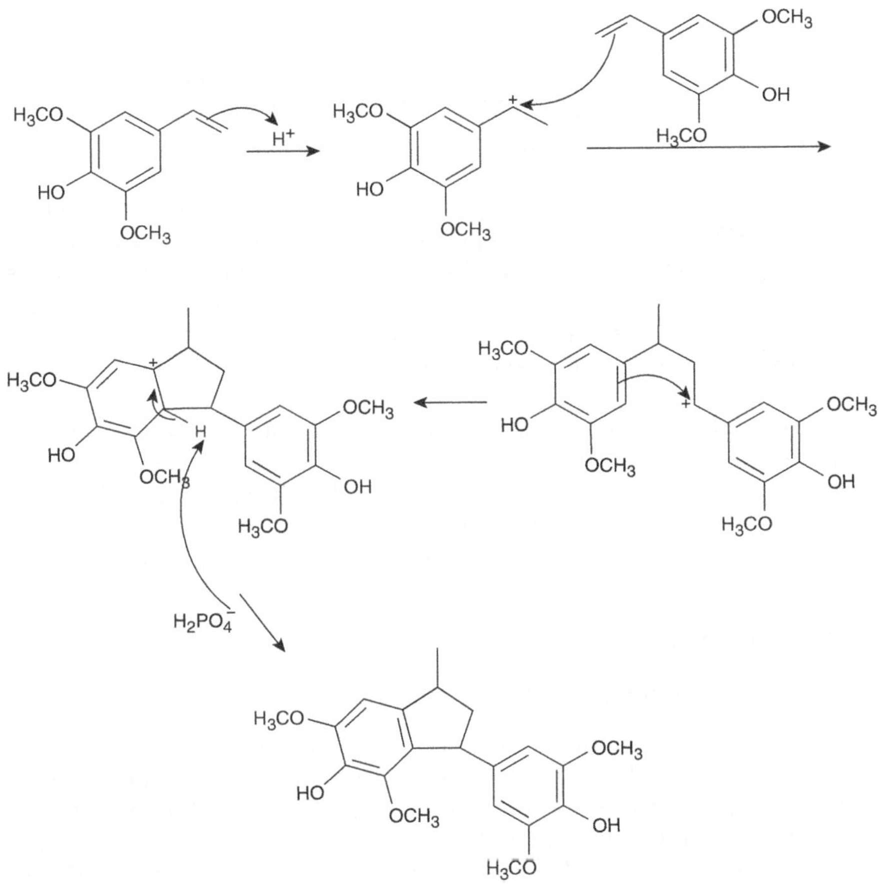

Figure 3.2 Recation mechanism for acid-catalyzed formation of 4-vinylsyringol dimer (Kraljić et al. 2015).

3.2 *Identification*

3.2.1 *Mass spectrometry*

The identification of 4-vinylsyringol monomer and its di- or trimers is mostly done by mass spectrometry. In electrospray ionization, the following masses are detected for 4-vinylsyringol monomer, di- and trimers in positive and negative modes, respectively: 180 ($[M+H]^+ = 181$) 360 ($[M+H]^- = 359$) and 540 ($[M+H]^- = 539$). In addition, the parent ions can be fragmented multiple times in ion trap MS, yielding a range of characteristic fragments (cf. 3.3; Harbaum-Piayda et al. 2010).

3.2.2 NMR

The dimer of 4-vinylsyringol was isolated by preparative HPLC and the structure was elucidated by NMR. In the ^{13}C NMR and ^{1}H NMR spectra, two sets of nearly identical signals were detected in a ratio of 3 to 1, respectively, suggesting that it is a mixture of two diastereomers (Harbaum-Piayda et al. 2010; Kraljić et al. 2015). To further determine the structure, various NMR experiments were performed to assign C- and H-atoms and to reveal the respective vicinities by visualizing H-H and C-C couplings. The two vinylsyringol monomers enter into a substituted indane linkage. In this case, the phenolic residue of a vinylsyringol monomer forms a phenolic substituent attached to the indane backbone via the C3-atom (Figure 3.2).

This position was confirmed by cross peaks of H-3 and C-2' and C-6' in NMR experiments. The binding is predominantly in cis-configuration and to a lesser extent in trans-configuration. Furthermore, there is a characteristic methyl group (C-8) in the indane skeleton that couples with the H1-atom as well as the C1a-atom (Harbaum-Piayda et al. 2010).

3.3 Quantification

3.3.1 Extraction and sample pretreatment

In recent years, different pretreatment methods have been developed to extract and purify phenolic components from oilseeds, oil, and side products. Among the most important methods are the liquid-liquid extraction (LLE), solid-liquid extraction and solid-phase extraction (SPE). Thin layer chromatography (TLC) (Wakamatsu et al. 2005) is also used in multistep sample preparation procedures, usually in conjunction with identification and structure elucidation. Furthermore, the following methods have been described for the extraction of phenolic compounds: dispersive liquid-liquid microextraction (DLLME) using ethanol:water 60:40 (v/v) as extracting solvent and 1,4-dioxane as disperser solvent (Godoy-Caballero et al. 2013). This method can be considered as a miniaturized version of conventional LLE consisting of a tenary system which requires only microliter volumes of solvents. In the conventional DLLME water-immiscible chlorinated solvents were used as extractants (Asensio-Ramos et al. 2011). Further, the following methods are in use for phenolic analysis: magnetic solid phase extraction (MSPE) (Wu et al. 2016) and supercritical fluid extraction (SFE) (Silva et al. 2019).

LLE of sinapic acid and vinylsyringol from oil is usually carried out with methanol or aqueous methanolic solutions. However, the extraction efficiency on monomers and dimers of 4-vinylsyringol varies.

Using pure methanol results in better extraction for both compounds compared to aqueous methanolic solutions (50/50), but the difference is higher for monomers than for dimers (Harbaum-Piayda et al. 2010). Hexane, heptane, and cyclohexane were selected as nonpolar solvents to isolate phenolic compounds from rapeseed lecithin. Subsequently, 70% ethanol (v/v) was used to extract twice to isolate the polar compounds. While the combined extraction (nonpolar solvent and 70% ethanol) yielded higher contents for sinapine and sinapic acid, single extraction (70% ethanol) yielded higher contents of 4-vinylsyringol (Harbaum-Piayda et al. 2010).

With the accelerated extraction method, extraction of rapeseed meal is performed at elevated temperatures (140°C–180°C) and increased pressure (1500 psi). Sieved samples were mixed with Ottawa sand at a ratio of 1:5 to optimize extraction efficiency; several cycles can be performed with fresh solvent-water mixtures (30%–70% solvent fraction). The highest yield of phenolic compounds was obtained when 70% methanol or 70% ethanol is used at a temperature of 180°C (Nandasiri et al. 2021a, 2021b). The recovery is 85%–91% when the samples are spiked with sinapic acid.

A simple and rapid enrichment technique is solid-phase extraction (SPE) for routine analysis of phenolic constituents in oils. For example, C8-, C18-, and diol-cartridges are used to extract phenolic acids, phenolic alcohols, flavonoids, and secoiridoids from oils. Siger et al. (2017) applied this method for the extraction of phenols (including 4-vinylsyringol) from rapeseed oil. The main drawback of these SPE methods is the pre– or post–SPE procedure for the reconstituted extracts, the lyophilized crude oilseeds, or the concentration of the oil fractions.

Recently, a novel mixed-mode and ion-exchange adsorbent was developed for the purification and enrichment of low-concentration polar compounds in oils by ionic species and effective retention of uncharged species by hydrophobic and hydrophilic interactions (Yu et al. 2021).

3.3.2 Chromatographic separation

For liquid chromatic separation by HPLC, reverse solid phases based on C8- or C18-modified silica gel particles are mainly used. Gradient systems are usually employed for elution and, less frequently, chromatography is isocratic (Table 3.1). The gradient systems mostly consist of two eluents that alternate in their proportions over the chromatography time. At the start of chromatography, the aqueous eluent has the highest proportion, and as chromatography proceeds, the proportion of the second eluent, which consists of methanol, acetonitrile, or a mixture of the two, is gradually increased. Phosphoric, formic, or acetic acid are added to the aqueous

Table 3.1 Methods for quantification of sinapic acid, canolol (4-vinylsyringo) and its dimer

	Extraction/ injection	Solid phase	Eluents	Gradient	Detectionmode (ionisation mode)	Retention times	Author
1	1 g **oil**/9 mL solvent (methanol/ water 70:30, v/v) 3 times and made up to 25 mL 0.2 g **Protein** 3 times and made up to 10 mL	RP Phenomenex (250 × 4.6 mm)	A: water/methanol (90:10, v/v) with 1.2% o-phosphoric acid as B: methanol (100%) with 0.1% o-phosphoric acid	0, 7, 20, 25, and 28 min with 10, 20, 45, 70 and 100% B with a post-run of 10 min.	UV: 275 nm sinapic acid; 330 nm vinylsyringol (not detected)		Thiyam et al. (2006), Thiyam et al. (2009)
2		RP Phenomenex Synergi Fusion (125 × 3 mm)	A Water (5 mmL/l ammonium acetate buffer adjusted to pH 3.2 with acetic acid) B MeOH	0,7,20,25,28,30,33,40 with A 90, 80, 55, 30, 0, 0, 90 and 90%	MS (Ion Trap) Scna mode 150–600; fragmentation energy 30% ESI spray voltage 3.5 kV		Thiyam et al. (2009)
3	No information about extraction procedure 3µl	Acquity BEH Shield RP18 (100 × 2.1 mm, 1.7 µm)	A 2% actic acid (w/w) B 100 MeOH	5%–25% B (7.40 min), 25%–29% B (2.67 min), 29%–36% B (6.66 min), 36%–45% B (6.67 min), 45%–65% B (2 min), 45%–65% B (2 min), 65%–5% B (2 min), and 5% B (2.67 min).	PDA 270 nm for 4-vinylsyringol and 330 nm for the other compounds		Yu et al. (2020)

4	**Oil**; SPE diol (500 mg) (Supelco) conditioning the column (5 mL MeOH, 5 mL n-hexane); adding the samples (2.5 g oil in 5 mL n-hexane and 5 mL n-hexane); washing (5 mL n--hexane/ethyl acetate 90:10 v/v); eluting MeOH 5 mL	LiChrosorb Si 60 column (250 × 4.6 mm, 5 µm) from Merck (Darmstadt, Germany)	n-hexane with 1,4-dioxane (96:4 v/v)	isocratic	fluorescence 4-vinylsyringol excitation 280 nm and emission 325 nm.	Siger et al. (2017)
5	Extracts from Meal (accelerated solvent extraction)	Kinetex RP Biphenyl C18 100 Å RP column (2.6 mm, 150 × 4.6 mm) Phenomenex	A 0.1% (v/v) formic acid B MeOH [0.1% (v/v) formic acid]	B: 25%–25% B (0–3 min), 25%–40% (3–8 min), 40%–40% (8–13 min), 40%–60% (13–25 min), 60%–70% (25–38 min), 70%–100% (38–41 min), 100%–100% (41–44 min), 100%–25% (44–47 min), and 25%–25% (47–57 min)	MS ESI, positive Mass range 50–2500 m/z 3.5 kV 200°C $[M+H]^+$ 181.1 4-vinylsyringol Sinapine: $[M+H]^+$ 310.15	Nandasiri et al. (2021a)

(Continued)

Table 3.1 (Continued)

	Extraction/ injection	Solid phase	Eluents	Gradient	Detectionmode (ionisation mode)	Retention times	Author
6	Extracts from Meal (accelerated solvent extraction)	Kinetex RP Biphenyl C18 100 Å RP column (2.6 mm, 150 × 4.6 mm) Phenomenex	A 0.1% (v/v) formic acid B MeOH [0.1% (v/v) formic acid]	B: 25%–25% B (0–3 min), 25%–40% (3–8 min), 40%–40% (8–13 min), 40%–60% (13–25 min), 60%–70% (25–38 min), 70%–100% (38–41 min), 100%–100% (41–44 min), 100%–25% (44–47 min), and 25%–25% (47–57 min)	DAD 270 nm (4-vinylsyringol) and 330 nm (sinapine and sinapic acid)		Nandasiri et al. (2019)
7	Hexane, heptane, and cyclohexane combined wiht 70% EtOH Direct extraction with 70% EtOH	SUPELCOSIL LC-18 (a 25 cm 4.6 mm, 5 mm)	A (0.08 mol/L KH2PO4:CH3CN:85% H3PO4 (85:15:0.25) B (60% MeOH: 85%H3PO4 (100:0.05))	t0–t18 100% A, t23–t320%A, and t37–t42100%A	HPLC-DAD sinapine and sinapic acid were detected at 330 nm; while 4-vinylsyringol was detected at 270 nm.	13 Sinapine 15 Sinapic Acid 27 4-vinylsyringol	Li und Guo (2016)
8	5 µL sample	SB C18 column (RRHD, 2.1 × 50 mm; 1.8 µm)	A: 0.1% acetic acid in methanol B: aqueous 0.1% acetic acid.	0 min 0% A; 1.5 min 45% A, 4 min 70% A 6.5 min 80% A, 7.5 min 90% A, 7.6–10 min, 10% A.	MRM; (ESI)	Sinapic acid Sinapine Sinapolyglucosides 4-vinylsyringol	Yu et al. (2021)
9		RP 18	A 0.2% phosphoric acid B MeOH C ACN	Terner Gradient ABC (%/%/%) 0 min 96/2/2 40 min 50/25/25 45 min 40/30/30 60 min 0/50/50 70 min 0/50/50	Tripelquadrupole $[M+Na]^+$ 203.1 (4-vinylsyringol) and 383.2 (Dimer 4-vinylsyringol)		Kraljić et al. (2019)

10	Oil, Deodestillate (2 g) 3 mL MeOH Oil, Deodestillate (10 g) in 10 mL hexane disssolved, extraction with 50% aquous MeOH	C-8 Chrospher (250 × 4 mm, 5 µm)	A 0.1% formic acid B MeOH	5 min 30% B 15 min 50% B 20 min 90% B 29 min 100% B 30 min 30% B 35 min 30% B	DAD 280 nm Trap ESI $[M+H]^+$ 181 m/z $[M+H]^-$ 359 m/z Dimer 4-vinylsyringol $[M+H]^-$ 539 m/z Trimer 4-vinylsyringol	13.4 min 20.8 min 21.6 min	Harbaum-Piayda et al. (2010)
11	Oil; extraction with MeOH, 2 times, dried with N2 and reconstituted in MeOH	BEH C18 (100 × 2.1 mm; 1.7 µm)	A acetic acid 0.1% in water B MeOH	0–0.5 min 99% [A] 0.5–4.5 min 30% [A], 4.5–5.5 min 10% [A], 5.5–6 min 99% [A]	Single Quadrupol No further information	4-vinylsyringol 4.27 min	McDowell et al. (2017)
12	Rapseeds Alkaline hydrolysis, extract mixed with dest. H_2O und 1.5 mL 10 M NaOH, pH adjusted to 2 with 8 M HCl, extraction with 3 mL ethyl acetate (3x), dried unter N2, reconstituted with 5 mL MeOH und 15 mL 0.2§ acetic acid.	Zorbax Eclipse Plus C18 (2.1 × 150 mm; 1.8 µm)	A acetic acid 0.2% in water (v/v) B MeOH	0–5 min 20–40% B 6 min 40% B 7 min 40–50% B 8 min 50% B 13 min 50–60% B 15 min 60–70% B 16 min 70% B 17 min 70–20% B 22 min 20%	DAD 330 nm SA 280 nm 4-vinylsyringol	9.5 min SA 14.4 min 4-vinylsyringol	Shrestha et al. (2012)

(*Continued*)

Table 3.1 (Continued)

	Extraction/ injection	Solid phase	Eluents	Gradient	Detectionmode (ionisation mode)	Retention times	Author
13	2 g **Oil** dissolved in hexane	Nucleolsil 100 NH2 (150 × 4 mmm, 5 μm)	Hexane/Isopropanol (96:4 v/v)	Isocratic	UV 275	4-vinylsyringol 6.8 min	Spielmeyer et al. (2009)
14	Oil	Luna NH2 100 column (250 × 4.6 mm i.d., particle size 5 μm) Phenomenex	Hexane:isopropanol (96:4 v/v)	Isocratic	Fluorescence excitation/ emission 290/330 nm		Cortese et al. (2019)
15							Chew (2020)

Note: MRM, multiple reaction monitoring; DAD, Diode Array Detection; PDA, photodiode array.

phase, with formic and acetic acid being used primarily when the chromatography unit is coupled to a mass spectrometer.

Retention occurs upon separation on a reverse solid phase in the order of sinapic acid, 4-vinylsyringol, and dimer and trimer of vinylsyringol. Retention times ranged from 29.12 (sinapic acid) to 51.54 (dimer) in the study by (Kraljić et al. 2015) and from 9.1 to 21.6 (trimer) in the study by Harbaum-Piayda et al. (2010) (Figure 3.3).

With respect to sinapic acid, the following retention factors are calculated: for 4-vinylsyringol 1.45 (Kraljić et al. 2015) and 1.47 (Harbaum-Piayda et al. 2010), for the dimer 1.77 (Kraljić et al. 2015) and 2.28 (Harbaum-Piayda et al. 2010), and for the trimer 2.37 (Harbaum-Piayda et al. 2010).

Normal phase chromatography is less frequently used in studies. However, it has the advantage that oil dissolved in solvent can be analyzed directly if the concentrations are high enough. Normal phase chromatography separates 4-vinylsyringol among the phenolic compounds in rapeseed, as well as tocopherols in one run (Siger et al. 2017).

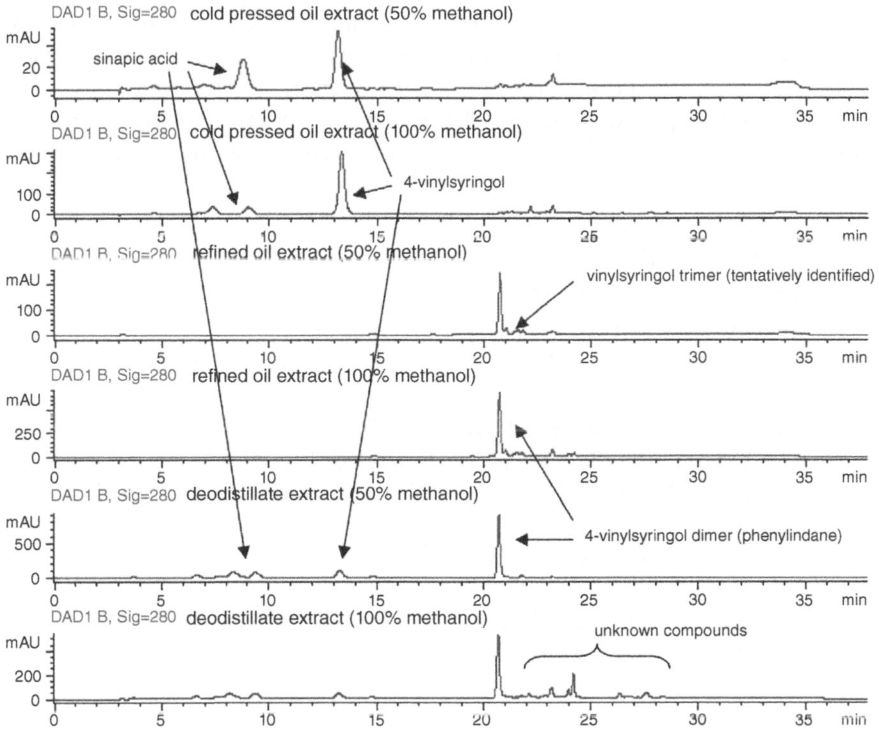

Figure 3.3 HPLC–chromatograms of extracts (Harbaum-Piayda et al. 2010).

3.3.3 Detection

The detection of 4-vinylsyringol is usually done together with sinapic acid, since their occurrence in oil and side-stream products is related to each other. In UV detection, vinylsyringol and its dimers or trimers are quantified at 280 nm, while hydroxycinnamic acid is usually quantified at 330 nm. The difference in maxima is due to the fact that the typical trans-double bond to the carboxyl group of the cinnamic acids changes to a vinyl group during the formation of vinylsyringol by decarboxylation. In contrast, the phenol group responsible for the absorption at 280 nm is retained. 4-Vinylsyringol exhibits absorption peaks at 218 and 269 nm. The molecular extinction coefficient in water was reported by Wakamatsu et al. (2005) as 29,000 at 218 nm and 13,000 at 269 nm (εmol/l; 1 cm).

Compared with the sensitivity and specificity, tandem mass spectrometry is the predominant platform for the analysis of trace amounts of phenolic compounds in oil matrix. Different mass spectrometer types are used for analysis and identification, such as triple quadrupole detector, ion trap detector, and less commonly single quadrupole for quantification (Table 3.1). For identification, characteristic fragment ions are important in addition to molecular mass. When using an ion trap as a detector, multiple fragmentations up to MS^6 for the dimer and MS^8 for the trimer can be made. These are described below for compounds with different mass spectrometers, since the compounds are currently not commercially available. For ion trap and triple quadrupole mass spectrometers, the following mass values with the corresponding intensities were reported in the literature:

Ion trap mass spectrometer:

- 4-Vinylsyringol $[M+H]^+$ = 181
  MS^2 $[M+H]^+$ 150 (8), 149 (100), 121 (12), 93 (3)
  MS^3 [MS^2 (149 m/z)] 121 (100), 103 (6), 93 (51) (Harbaum-Piayda et al. 2010)
- Dimer of 4-vinylsyringol $[M-H]^-$ =359
  MS^2 $[M-H]^-$ 345 (2), 344 (100), 329 (8), 152(3)
  MS^3 [MS^2 (344 m/z)] 344 (2) 329 (100), 192 (3), 177 (3), 152 (4) (Harbaum-Piayda et al. 2010)
- Trimer of 4-vinylsyringol $[M-H]^-$ = 539
  MS^2 $[M-H]^-$ 524 (100), 522 (17), 509 (8)
  MS^3 [MS^2 (524 m/z)] 509 (25), 508 (30), 507 (100), 357 (8), 355 (8), 343 (12) (Harbaum-Piayda et al. 2010)

Triplequadrupol mass spectrometer:

4-Vinylsyringol: $[M+Na]^+$= 203,1, main fragment ions: 181, 149, 121 (Kraljić et al. 2015)

4-Vinylsyringol: $[M+H]^+$=181 (64) main fragment ions: 166 (16), 149 (100), 121 (84), 103 (54), 93 (66), 77 (15) (Spielmeyer et al. 2009)
4-Vinylsyringol-dimer: $[M+Na]^+$=383.2 H main fragment ions: 207.2, 175.2, 147.1, 143.1, 132.1, 129.1, 119.1, 115.1, 107.2, 91.2 (Kraljić et al. 2015)

3.3.4 Derivatization and labeling

Simultaneous quantification is not always satisfactory for numerous phenolic compounds by LC-MS/MS at low concentrations due to low ionization efficiency. In addition, matrix effects associated with endogenous lipids occur in the measurement. This can lead to larger deviations in quantification without the use of stable isotope-labeled internal standards (Yu et al. 2021).

To improve the ionization efficiency and matrix effect, stable isotope dilution analysis has been developed and used for the accurate determination of phenolic compounds in biological and plant samples. However, phenolic compounds labeled with stable isotopes are very difficult to synthesize. Therefore, chemical labeling by stable isotope-labeled groups of phenolic compounds is an interesting alternative method. Chemical labeling of polyphenols can be done with deuterated dansyl chloride (d_6-DnCl). Dansyl chlorides (d_0-dansyl chloride, d_0-DnCl) and d_6-DnCl react with the polyphenolic extract and standard substances, respectively. Due to the change in physicochemical properties after dansylation, the labeled phenolic compounds not only have good affinity for the C18 solid phase and improved chromatographic separation, but the introduction of the tertiary amino group also enhances the signal intensity in mass spectrometry (Yu et al. 2021).

Rapeseed phenolic compounds $[M + H]^+$ were readily protonated, forming fragment ions at m/z 171.1 and 156.2 (d_0-DnCl phenolic compound) and 177.1 (d_6-DnCl phenolic compound). Each ion pair was consistently detectable with a 6-Da mass shift between analytes and internal standards. Assignment and accurate quantification of phenolic compounds is possible in this manner. For sinapic acid, the following precursor and production (m/z) were detected: d_6-DnCl: 463.90 and 177.20 and d0-DnCl: 457.90, 171.20 and 156.2. For 4-vinylsyringol, the following precursor and production (m/z) were detected: d_6-DnCl: 420.2 and 177.10 and d_0-DnCl: 414.20, 171.10 and 156.15 (Yu et al. 2021).

3.3.5 Standards

For quantification, sinapic acid can be used as a commercial standard and the concentration of its derivatives is expressed in sinapine equivalents.

If 4-vinylsysringol is to be used as a standard substance, the compound must be synthesized or isolated. The synthesis can be done with two different starting substances, 4-acetoxy-3,5-dimethosystyrene or syringaldehyde.

When 4-acetoxy-3,5-dimethoxystyrene is used, proceed as follows. Dissolve 250 mg KOH in 1.25 mL methanol and then add to a solution of 250 mg 4-acetoxy-3,5-demethoxystyrene in 1.5 mL methanol and store overnight at room temperature. Then 250 μL of acetic acid is added to the solution and extracted three times with 5 mL of ethyl acetate. The collected organic phase is washed with 2.5 mL of water and 2.5 mL of 5% $NaHCO_3$ solution. The organic phase is removed under vacuum and purified by preparative HPLC. An RP-18 column (250 × 21 mm, 5 μm particle size) was used for this purpose. Two eluents (100% water and 100% methanol) were pumped as a gradient at a rate of 20 mL/min. The fraction after 4.5 to 5.5 min was collected and after removal of the eluent, a white powder was present with purity >99% as determined by HPLC-DAD-MS (Harbaum-Piayda et al. 2010).

Furthermore, the synthesis of vinylsyringol can be obtained from syringaldehyde as precursor (Rein et al. 2005). For this purpose, a Knoevenagel-Doebner condensation is carried out with malonic acid and piperidine in toluene at 115°C for 100 min. The yield is 47% (Simpson et al. 2005; Zago et al. 2016).

Alternatively, vinylsyringol can be obtained from a hexane/isopropanol extract by extracting three times with 0.1 M hydrochloric acid solution. Solid phase extraction (Chromabond HR-P) can be used to isolate vinylsyringol from the aqueous solution. Vinylsyringol was eluted with methanol and the eluate was again extracted with hexane. The hexane extracts were concentrated and purified by thin layer chromatography (silica gel 60, Merck, Germany) with a hexane/ethyl acetate mixture (7:3 v/v). The band observed under UV light (Rf 0.21) is extracted with chloroform (Spielmeyer et al. 2009).

The dimer of vinyl syringol can be obtained as a standard from rapeseed oil deodistillate due to its high concentration. For this purpose, the same preparative HPLC separation as for vinyl syringol is used. The deodestillate is dissolved in 50% aqueous methanol. The fraction eluting after 6–7 min is collected and freeze dried (Harbaum-Piayda et al. 2010).

3.4 *Formation of canolol (4-vinylsyringol) dimers and fate of sinapic acid and monomers of canolol during rapeseed processing*

Although high levels of sinapic acid and sinapine are found in rapeseed, they are only present in small amounts in cold-pressed oil and are no longer found in refined edible oils. This is mainly due to their polarity or water solubility. In contrast, 4-vinylsyringol as well as the dimer and trimer have a lower polarity and thus a tendency to pass into the oil phase during processing.

3.4.1 *Crude oil and cold pressed oil*

During the processing of rapeseed, the next step is the formation of 4-vinylsyringol, so that significant amounts already occur in the pressed rapeseed oil, but the dimer is present in traces or not detectable. Kraljić et al. (2015) studied two batches and detected 0.3–0.6 mg/kg dimers and 229.7–375.2 mg/kg monomers of vinylsyringol in pressed crude oil. Harbaum-Piayda et al. (2010) detected dimers in 2 out of 6 cold-pressed rapeseed oils (max. 10.4 mg/kg) and 4-vinylsyringol monomer content ranged from 2.36 to 42.5 mg/kg. Here it can be assumed that different temperatures during pressing led to the differences and only at elevated temperatures, which are applied for pressing crude oil for raffinates, dimerization occurs. The absence of dimers in pressed rapeseed oil could be used as a quality criterion for gentle pressing of rapeseed. In contrast, Kraljić et al. (2015) found that dimerization does not occur when crude oil is heated to 95°C. So here it seems to be crucial that the heating takes place before or during pressing and not only in the isolated oil.

3.4.2 *Microwave treatment*

Microwave treatment has been reported in recent years as a promising method for rapeseed, resulting in the degradation of sinapic acid to 4-vinylsyringol.

Rapeseed roasting has been tested to determine the optimal formation of vinylsyringol. Spielmeyer et al. (2009) used different treatment times by heating the canola seed in the microwave at 800 watts for 1.5 min each time. From 1 to 6 cycles were applied and temperatures in the canola seed increased to 73°C–161°C. Longer heating time also increased the vinyl syringol content from 5.8 in the starting material to 703.2 µg/g. After the 4th cycle, a temperature of 135°C was reached and the concentration jumped from 54.4 to 340 µg/g of canola seed. The highest level was reached after 5 cycles and a total heating time of 7.5 min. A longer microwave treatment resulted in lower levels.

Cong et al. (2020) studied 39 different varieties and investigated the levels of sinapic acid derivatives and vinyl syringol before and after microwave treatment. While 4-vinylsyringol did not occur in the control sample, the content after microwave treatment ranged from 6.16 to 76.1 mg/100 g. There was a decrease in all sinapic acid derivatives. The decrease in sinapic acid alone could not have explained the amount of 4-vinylsyringol formed, so the authors assumed that sinapic acid derivatives also contributed to the formation of 4-vinylsyringol. The formation of dimers or trimers was not reported in either study. Based on the methodological data for analysis, it can be suspected that the dimers or trimers may be present but were not detected chromatographically.

3.5 Neutralization

Kraljić et al. (2015) investigated the formation of 4-vinylsyringol dimers during the neutralization process. First, phosphoric acid was added and subsequently neutralized with NaOH. They found that the addition of phosphoric acid played an important role and that only in its presence there was an increase in the content of dimers with a simultaneous decrease in monomeric 4-vinylsyringol. Depending on how much phosphoric acid was used, there was a loss of polyphenols between 21% and 63% and the content of dimers increased from 0.6 to 5.5 mg/kg and from 0.3 to 29.8 mg/kg of oil, respectively. The addition of NaOH resulted equally in the degradation of monomers and dimers. This supported their proposed mechanism, namely that the process of dimerization is acid catalyzed.

3.5.1 Bleaching

During bleaching, there is also a significant decrease in 4-vinylsyringol. At high initial 4-vinylsyringol content (after neutralization), there was an increase in dimers (from 6.6 to 18.3 mg/kg), while in oil with low initial content, the content of dimers decreased (from 29.8 to 20.8 mg/kg) (Kraljić et al. 2015).

3.5.2 Deodorization

Analysis of a deodistillate produced in the commercial refining process showed that polyphenols are transferred to a large extent into the distillate and there is a strong enrichment. 3.5 g/kg of dimers and 226 mg/kg of 4-vinylsyringol were found. In comparison, the content of tocopherols was only 22 mg/kg, while in the refined oil the contents were between 581 and 650 mg/kg (Harbaum-Piayda et al. 2010).

3.6 Metabolome

The analysis of all small molecules (metabolites) with a molecular weight of <1500 Da is called metabolomics analysis. The masses of metabolites found are matched with entries in databases and an abundance of metabolites can be assigned. In a study by Yang et al. (2019), 152 metabolites were found in rapeseed from three different origins. Among them, were sinapine and sinapic acid. The authors explained the occurrence of 4-vinylsyringol with the processing conditions, which is consistent with other studies. However, 4-vinylsyringol was not among the metabolites the authors found in the metabolomic analyses. They observed that there were clear differences based on metabolite profile between Canada, China, and Mongolia. It was shown that higher levels of sinapine and sinapic acid occurred in rapeseed in China than in Canada. Thus, Chinese rapeseed oil has a significant potential for the formation of 4-vinylsyringol in edible oil.

References

Aldabalde, V, Derrudi, M, Gamenara, D, Geymonat, F, Saenz-Méndez, P, Risso, M, Seoane, G (2011) Organocatalyzed decarboxylation of naturally occurring cinnamic acids. potential role in flavoring chemicals production. *Open Journal of Physical Chemistry* 01 (03), 85–93. DOI: 10.4236/ojpc.2011.13012

Asensio-Ramos, M, Ravelo-Pérez, LM, González-Curbelo, M, Hernández-Borges, J (2011) Liquid phase microextraction applications in food analysis. *Journal of Chromatography: A* 1218 (42), 7415–7437. DOI: 10.1016/j.chroma.2011.05.096

Bernini, R, Mincione, E, Barontini, M, Provenzano, G, Setti, L (2007) Obtaining 4-vinylphenols by decarboxylation of natural 4-hydroxycinnamic acids under microwave irradiation. *Tetrahedron* 63 (39), 9663–9667.

Chew, S (2020) Cold-pressed rapeseed (*Brassica napus*) oil: Chemistry and functionality. *Food Research International (Ottawa, Ont.)* 131, 108997. DOI: 10.1016/j.foodres.2020.108997

Cong, Y, Zheng, M, Huang, F, Liu, C, Zheng, C (2020) Sinapic acid derivatives in microwave-pretreated rapeseeds and minor components in oils. *Journal of Food Composition and Analysis* 87, 103394. DOI: 10.1016/j.jfca.2019.103394

Cortese, CM., Portela, G, Sánchez, RJ, Fernández, MB (2019) Improving the canolol amount and the yield of expressed canola oil applying combined pretreatments. *International Food Research Journal* 26 (1): 99–104.

Fiddler, W, Parker, W, Wasserman, AE, Doerr, RC (1967) Thermal decomposition of ferulic acid. *Journal of Agricultural and Food Chemistry* 15 (5), 757–761.

Frank, O, Blumberg, S, Kunert, C, Zehentbauer, G, Hofmann, T (2007) Structure determination and sensory analysis of bitter-tasting 4-vinylcatechol oligomers and their identification in roasted coffee by means of LC-MS/MS. *Journal of Agricultural and Food Chemistry* 55 (5), 1945–1954.

Godoy-Caballero, MP, Acedo-Valenzuela, MI, Galeano-Díaz, T (2013) New reversed phase dispersive liquid-liquid microextraction method for the determination of phenolic compounds in virgin olive oil by rapid resolution liquid chromathography with ultraviolet-visible and mass spectrometry detection. *Journal of Chromatography: A* 1313, 291–301. DOI: 10.1016/j.chroma.2013.06.020

Harbaum-Piayda, B, Oehlke, K, Sönnichsen, FD., Zacchi, P, Eggers, R, Schwarz, K (2010) New polyphenolic compounds in commercial deodistillate and rapeseed oils. *Food Chemistry* 123 (3), 607–615. DOI: 10.1016/j.foodchem.2010.04.078

Koski, A, Pekkarinen, S, Hopia, A, Wähälä, K, Heinonen, M (2003) Processing of rapeseed oil: Effects on sinapic acid derivative content and oxidative stability. *European Food Research and Technology* 217 (2), 110–114.

Kraljić, K, Brkan, V, Škevin, D, Srček, V, Radošević, K (2019) Canolol Dimer, a biologically active phenolic compound of edible rapeseed oil. *Lipids* 54 (2–3), 189–200. DOI: 10.1002/lipd.12132

Kraljić, K, Škevin, D, Barišić, L, Kovačević, M, Obranović, M, Jurčević, I (2015) Changes in 4-vinylsyringol and other phenolics during rapeseed oil refining. *Food Chemistry* 187, 236–242. DOI: 10.1016/j.foodchem.2015.04.039

Kuwahara, H, Kanazawa, A, Wakamatu, D, Morimura, S, Kida, K, Akaike, T, Maeda, H (2004) Antioxidative and antimutagenic activities of 4-vinyl-2,6-dimethoxyphenol (canolol) isolated from canola oil. *Journal of Agricultural and Food Chemistry* 52 (14), 4380–4387. DOI: 10.1021/jf040045+

Li, J, Guo, Z (2016) Identification and quantification of phenolic compounds in rapeseed originated lecithin and antioxidant activity evaluation. *LWT* 73 (7), 397–405. DOI: 10.1016/j.lwt.2016.06.039

Liu, Q, Wu, L, Pu, H, Li, C, Hu, Q (2012) Profile and distribution of soluble and insoluble phenolics in Chinese rapeseed (*Brassica napus*). *Food Chemistry* 135 (2), 616–622. DOI: 10.1016/j.foodchem.2012.04.142

McDowell, D, Elliott, CT., Koidis, A (2017) Pre-processing effects on cold pressed rapeseed oil quality indicators and phenolic compounds. *European Journal of Lipid Science and Technology* 119 (9), 1600357. DOI: 10.1002/ejlt.201600357

Nandasiri, R, Eskin, NMA, Komatsu, E, Perreault, H, Thiyam-Holländer, U (2021a) Valorization of canola by-products: Concomitance of flavor-active bitter phenolics using pressurized heat treatments. *LWT* 138, 110397.

Nandasiri, R, Eskin, NAM, Thiyam-Höllander, U (2019) Antioxidative polyphenols of canola meal extracted by high pressure: Impact of temperature and solvents. *Journal of Food Science* 84 (11), 3117–3128. DOI: 10.1111/1750-3841.14799

Nandasiri, R, Imran, A, Thiyam-Holländer, U, Eskin, NAM (2021b) Rapidoxy® 100: A solvent-free pre-treatment for production of canolol. *Frontiers in Nutrition* 8, 687851. DOI: 10.3389/fnut.2021.687851

Oehlke, K, Harbaum-Piayda, B, Meyer, F, Eggers, R, Schwarz, K (2017) Antioxidant activity of deodorizer distillate fractions in rapeseed oil. *European Journal of Lipid Science and Technology* 119 (7), 1600273. DOI: 10.1002/ejlt.201600273

Rein, MJ., Ollilainen, V, Vahermo, M, Yli-Kauhaluoma, J, Heinonen, M (2005) Identification of novel pyranoanthocyanins in berry juices. *European Food Research and Technology* 220 (3-4), 239–244. DOI: 10.1007/s00217-004-1063-6

Shrestha, K, Stevens, CV, de Meulenaer, B (2012) Isolation and identification of a potent radical scavenger (canolol) from roasted high erucic mustard seed oil from Nepal and its formation during roasting. *Journal of Agricultural and Food Chemistry* 60 (30), 7506–7512. DOI: 10.1021/jf301738y

Siger, A, Józefiak, M, Górnaś, P (2017) Cold-pressed and hot-pressed rapeseed oil. The effects of roasting and seed moisture on the antioxi- dant activity, canolol, and tocopherol level. *Acta Scientiarum Polonorum: Technologia Alimentaria* 16 (1), 69–81. DOI: 10.17306/J.AFS.2017.0458

Siger, A, Nogala-Kalucka, M, Lampart-Szczapa, E (2008) The content and antioxidant activity of phenolic compounds in cold-pressed plant oils. *Journal of Food Lipids* 15 (2), 137–149. DOI: 10.1111/j.1745-4522.2007.00107.x

Silva, Lde O., Ranquine, LG., Monteiro, M, Torres, AG. (2019) Pomegranate (Punica granatum L.) seed oil enriched with conjugated linolenic acid (cLnA), phenolic compounds and tocopherols: Improved extraction of a specialty oil by supercritical CO_2. *The Journal of Supercritical Fluids* 147, 126–137.

Simpson, CJ, Fitzhenry, MJ, Stamford, N, Patrick J. (2005) Preparation of vinylphenols from 2- and 4-hydroxybenzaldehydes. *Tetrahedron Letters* 46 (40), 6893–6896. DOI: 10.1016/j.tetlet.2005.08.011

Spielmeyer, A, Wagner, A, Jahreis, G (2009) Influence of thermal treatment of rapeseed on the canolol content. *Food Chemistry* 112 (4), 944–948. DOI: 10.1016/j.foodchem.2008.07.011

Thiyam, U, Claudia, P, Jan, U, Alfred, B (2009) De-oiled rapeseed and a protein isolate. Characterization of sinapic acid derivatives by HPLC–DAD and LC–MS. *European Food Research and Technology* 229 (5), 825–831. DOI: 10.1007/s00217-009-1122-0

Thiyam, U, Stöckmann, H, Zum Felde, T, Schwarz, K (2006) Antioxidative effect of the main sinapic acid derivatives from rapeseed and mustard oil by-products. *European Journal of Lipid Science and Technology* 108 (3), 239–248.

Wakamatsu, D, Morimura, S, Sawa, T, Kida, K, Nakai, C, Maeda, H (2005) Isolation, identification, and structure of a potent alkyl-peroxyl radical scavenger in crude canola oil, canolol. *Bioscience, Biotechnology, and Biochemistry* 69 (8), 1568–1574. DOI: 10.1271/bbb.69.1568

Wu, R, Ma, F, Zhang, L, Li, P, Li, G, Zhang, Q et al. (2016) Simultaneous determination of phenolic compounds in sesame oil using LC-MS/MS combined with magnetic carboxylated multi-walled carbon nanotubes. *Food Chemistry* 204, 334–342. DOI: 10.1016/j.foodchem.2016.02.086

Yang, R, Deng, L, Zhang, L, Yue, X, Mao, J, Ma, F et al. (2019) Comparative metabolomic analysis of rapeseeds from three countries. *Metabolites* 9 (8). DOI: 10.3390/metabo9080161

Yu, G, Guo, T, Huang, Q (2020) Preparation of rapeseed oil with superhigh canolol content and superior quality characteristics by steam explosion pretreatment technology. *Food Science & Nutrition* 8 (5), 2271–2278. DOI: 10.1002/fsn3.1502

Yu, X, Yu, L, Ma, F, Li, P (2021) Quantification of phenolic compounds in vegetable oils by mixed-mode solid-phase extraction isotope chemical labeling coupled with UHPLC-MS/MS. *Food Chemistry* 334, 127572. DOI: 10.1016/j.foodchem.2020.127572

Zago, E, Dubreucq, E, Lecomte, J, Villeneuve, P, Fine, F, Fulcrand, H, Aouf, C (2016) Synthesis of bio-based epoxy monomers from natural allyl- and vinyl phenols and the estimation of their affinity to the estrogen receptor α by molecular docking. *New Journal of Chemistry* 40 (9), 7701–7710.

chapter four

Canolol production from a renewable feedstock via an engineered sinapic acid decarboxylase

Krista L. Morley

4.1 Introduction

The conversion of lignocellulosic biomass into biofuels and chemicals is a promising sustainable alternative to petroleum-based processes. Lignin is a major component of lignocellulosic biomass, in addition to cellulose and hemicellulose. In a biorefinery setting, lignin is considered to be a potential renewable source of aromatic chemicals (Kumar et al., 2021). Several approaches have been reported for the depolymerization of lignin to value-added products, including thermochemical (Hu et al., 2022), chemical catalysis (Bourbiaux et al., 2021; Abdelaziz et al., 2022), and biological (Fei Li et al., 2022; Weiland et al., 2022) methods. Another source of renewable aromatic compounds are plant cell wall polysaccharides esterified with hydroxycinnamic acids (HCAs). Hydroxycinnamic acids can be released from polysaccharides by employing alkaline hydrolysis (Sun et al., 2002) or phenolic acid esterases (Faulds and Williamson, 1995). Fruits, vegetables, and cereal grains are major dietary sources of HCAs (El-Seedi et al., 2012). The most abundant hydroxycinnamic acids found in nature are ferulic, caffeic, *p*-coumaric, and sinapic acid (Figure 4.1).

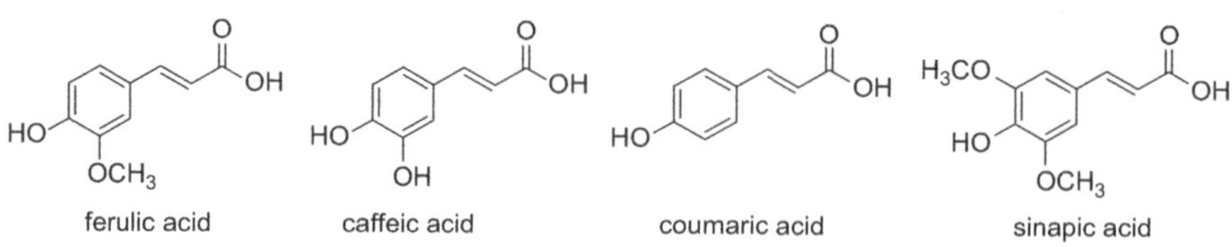

Figure 4.1 The chemical structures of ferulic, caffeic, coumaric, and sinapic acid.

DOI: 10.1201/b22828-4

Bioconversion of ferulic acid (FA) via microbial or enzymatic processes provide value-added products such as the flavoring agents vanillin (Rosazza et al., 1995), vinyl guaiacol (VG), (Huang et al., 1994), and 4-ethylguaiacol (Pesci et al., 2017). Several authors have reported on the enzymatic conversion of FA into VG using phenolic acid decarboxylase (PAD) enzymes. In addition, chemo-enzymatic routes have been reported for the conversion of FA to polyvinylguaiacol (PVG), a bio-based styrene alternative with desirable properties of biodegradability and strength (Leisch et al., 2013). Early reports describe the purification and characterization of PADs from *Bacillus pumilus* UI-670[1] (originally identified as *P. fluorescens*), *Bacillus pumilus* PS213 (Degrassi et al., 1995), *Bacillus subtilis* (Cavin et al., 1998), and *Lactobacillus plantarum* (Cavin et al., 1997). In addition, the PAD genes were cloned and expressed in *E. Coli* (Zago et al., 1995; Barthelmebs et al., 2001; Yang et al., 2009) and the recombinant enzymes were purified and characterized.

Substrate specificity studies determined that the PADs catalyzed the decarboxylation of 4-hydroxycinnamic acids, but not cinnamic or 2- and 3-hydroxycinnamic acids, thus indicating the requirement for a 4-hydroxy group in the substrate for the decarboxylation reaction to proceed (Figure 4.2).

To study the mechanism of decarboxylation, Rosazza and coworkers carried out deuterium-exchange studies with FA and the *P. fluorescens* PAD strain in an anaerobic environment. Based on the product analysis, the authors proposed that the decarboxylation of FA to VG proceeded via a non-oxidative mechanism involving an initial enzymatic isomerization of FA to a quinoid intermediate that spontaneously decarboxylates to yield the vinyl phenol (Figure 4.3) (Huang et al., 1993).

Since these preliminary mechanistic studies in the late 1990s, four crystal structures of PADs from *Lactobacillus plantarum* (2GC9) (Rodríguez et al., 2010), *Bacillus pumilus* UI-670 (3NAD) (Matte et al., 2010), *Enterobacter sp.* Px6-4 (3NX1) (Gu et al., 2011), and *Bacillus subtilis* (2P8G) (Frank et al., 2012), were published between 2009 and 2012. The four enzymes shared a

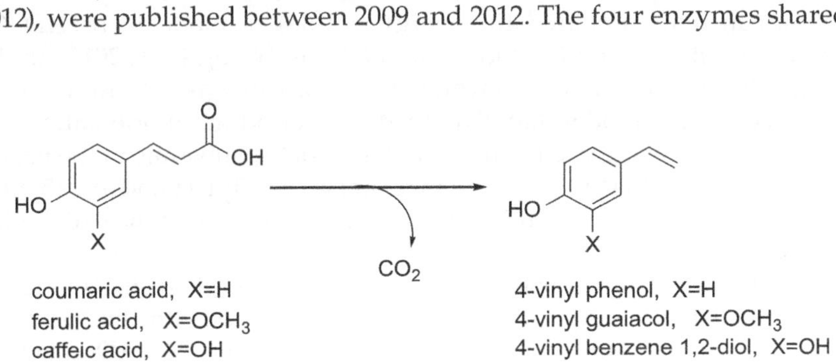

Figure 4.2 Reactions catalyzed by phenolic acid decarboxylases.

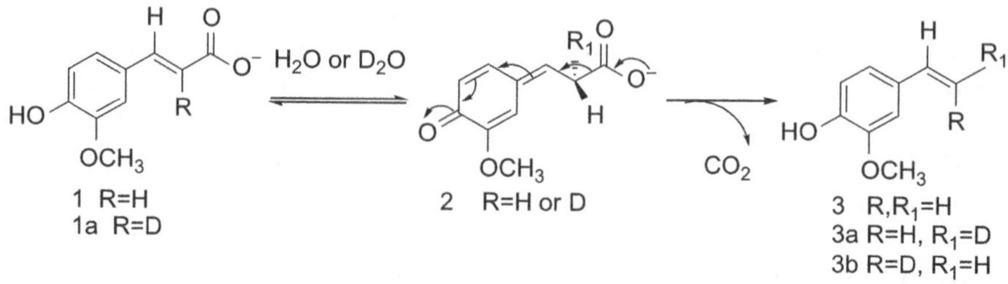

Figure 4.3 Proposed pathway for the biotransformation of ferulic acid by P. fluorescens.

(Adapted from Huang et al. (1993).

high level of amino acid sequence identity, and the crystal structures were superimposable. The four residues that were determined to be important for the activity of PAD from *L. plantarum* (LpPAD; Tyr18, Tyr20, Arg48 and Glu71) were structurally conserved between the four enzymes. Based on the mutational analysis of these active site residues, and in silico modeling of a complex of LpPAD and *p*-coumaric acid, Rodríguez et al. (2010) proposed a two-step catalytic mechanism in which the Glu71 residue acted as the catalytic base to deprotonate the *p*-hydroxy group of the substrate (Figure 4.4), and the Tyr18 and Tyr20 residues interacted with the carboxylate of the substrate to enable the release of CO_2.

The crystal structure of a complex of BsPAD Tyr19Ala mutant with *p*-coumaric acid revealed the substrate in an orientation that was consistent with the proposed mechanism based on the modeling of LpPAD (Rodríguez et al., 2010). In this complex structure, the Tyr11 and Tyr13 residues interacted with the carboxylate of *p*-coumaric acid and the phenolic hydroxy group of the substrate was H-bonded with the N atom of Arg41 (Figure 4.5) (Frank et al., 2012).

Later in 2015, a theoretical study was published on the PAD reaction mechanism that compared the energy profiles of modeled BsPAD–CA complexes with different substrate orientations (Sheng et al., 2015). In this study, the energetically most favorable mechanism was determined to be for the active-site model that contained CA bound in an orientation that was flipped 180° compared to the orientation of the substrate in the BsPAD crystal structure. In this proposed mechanism, the Tyr 11 and Tyr 13 interacted with the *p*-hydroxy group of the substrate instead of the carboxylate (Figure 4.6).

As described previously, most of the early mechanistic, modeling, and crystallization studies of PADs were performed with the substrates FA and CA (Huang et al., 1993). However, reports of the PAD-catalyzed decarboxylation of sinapic acid (SA, 3,5-dimethoxy-4-hydroxycinnamic acid) to 4-vinylsyringol (VS) were far less common (Hashidoko and Tahara,

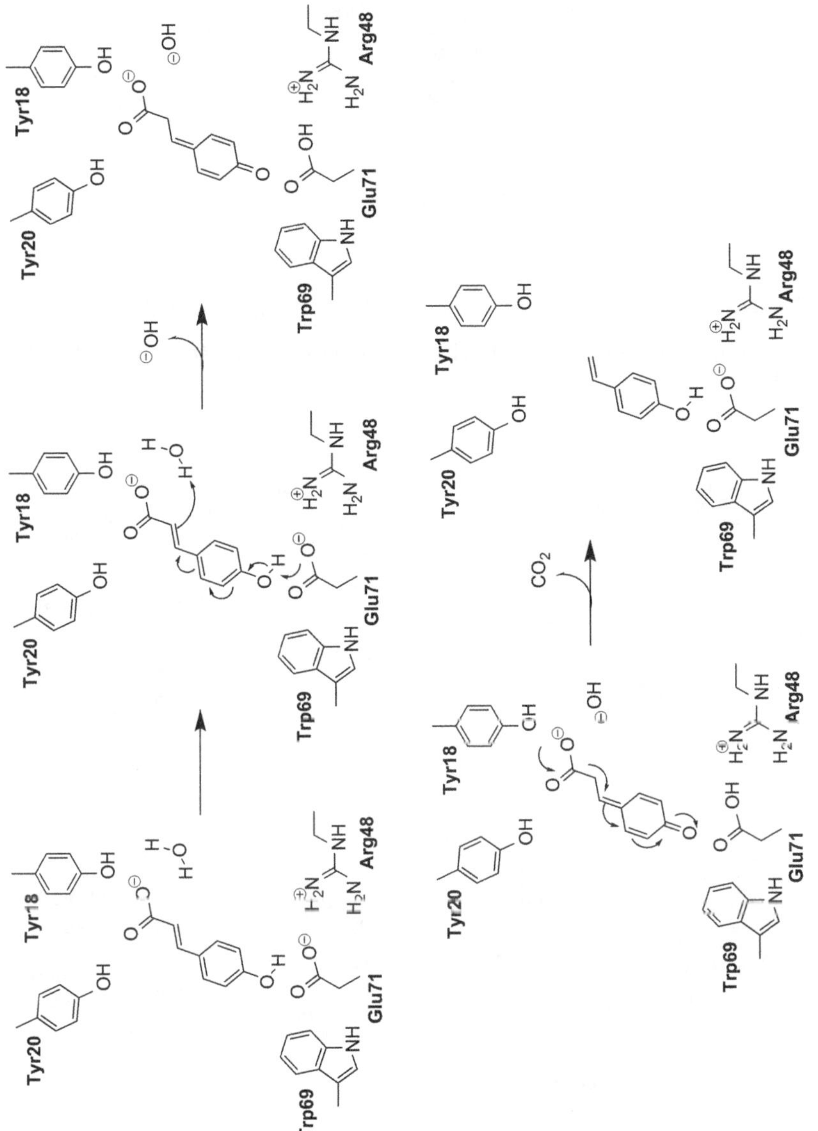

Figure 4.4 Proposed mechanism for the biotransformation of *p*-coumaric acid by LpPDC.
(Adapted from Rodríguez et al. (2010).

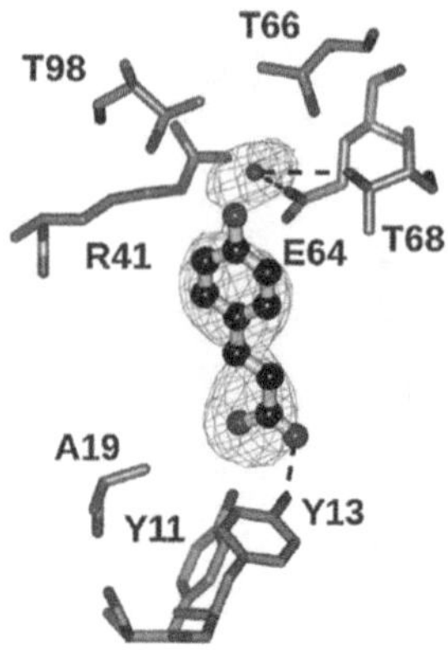

Figure 4.5 Active site of the Tyr19Ala mutant of BsPAD containing CA.

(Reprinted from Frank et al. (2012) with permission from Royal Society of Chemistry).

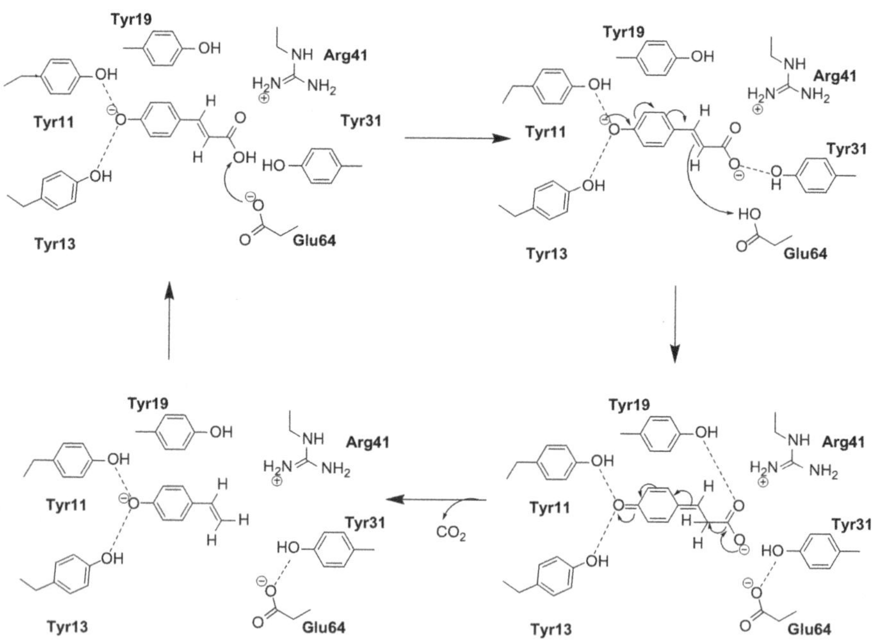

Figure 4.6 Proposed reaction mechanism of BsPAD.

(Adapted from Sheng et al. (2015).

1998). In comparison with FA, SA contains an additional methoxy group at the 5-position of the phenyl ring (Figure 4.7). SA has been identified in various fruits, vegetables, cereal grains, and oilseed crops (Nićiforović and Abramovič, 2014), and its esters are the major phenolic compounds in canola crops (Krygier et al., 1982; Naczk et al., 1998). Sinapine, the choline ester of sinapic acid, represents 70%–87% of the total phenolic content of different canola fractions. In one study that analyzed the extracts of canola seeds, press cakes, and meals, sinapine was reported to be in the ranges of 8.65–11.89, 9.90–11.31, and 6.11–10.11 mg/g, respectively (Khattab et al., 2010). In this same study, sinapoyl glucose, the glycoside derivative of sinapic acid, was reported in the ranges of 1.13 to 6.65, 2.37 to 4.01, and 1.35 to 1.99 mg/g in the extracts of canola seeds, press cakes, and meals, respectively. In comparison, the amount of free SA quantified in the three different fractions was less than 5% (0.8%–3.8%) and ranged between 0.09 and 0.59 mg/g.

SA, sinapine, and sinapoyl glucose all have significant antioxidative properties and their biological properties have been reported by several authors (Wanasundrara et al., 1994; Thiyam et al., 2006; Chen, 2016). Roasting of canola seeds leads to the formation of VS, another derivative of SA with antioxidant activity, antimutagenic (Kuwahara et al., 2004) anti-inflammatory, and anticarcinogenic properties (Cao et al., 2008). This compound was first isolated from crude canola oil and given the name canolol by Wakamatsu et al. (2005). In one study, the optimum roasting temperature for VS formation in canola seeds was determined to be 160°C and higher temperatures led to a reduction of the canolol content (Spielmeyer et al., 2009). Canolol is removed from canola oil during the refining process; however it can be re-added to frying oils to improve

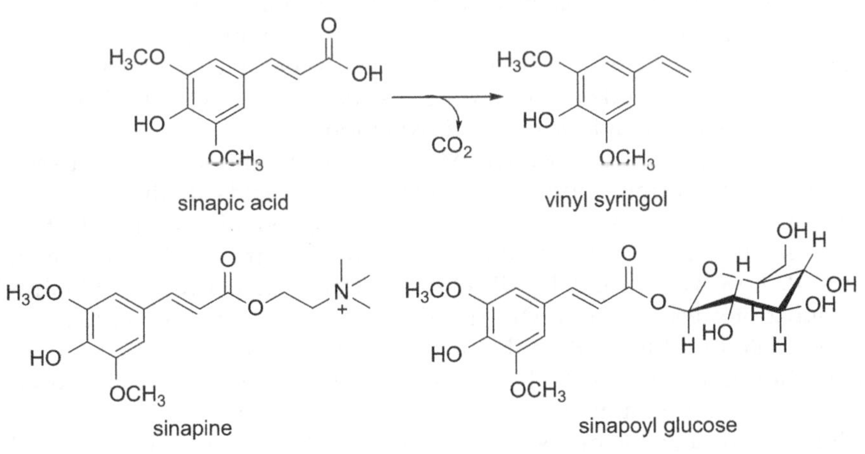

Figure 4.7 Sinapic acid, 4-vinylsyringol, sinapine, and sinapoyl glucose (Morley et al., 2013).

oxidative stability (Aachary et al., 2014). In addition, canolol can be used as a bio-based monomer in the preparation of bisphenol A analogues (Zago et al., 2016) and thermoplastic biopolymers.

Besides its extraction from crude canola oil, several chemical routes have been reported for the preparation of VS. VS can be synthesized by thermal- or microwave-induced decarboxylation of SA in the presence of a base catalyst (Nakamura et al., 1986; Bernini et al., 2007; Sharma et al., 2008; Terpinc et al., 2011), and a catalyst-free decarboxylation of SA at 170°C in DMF has also been reported. (Yang et al., 2022). Starting from syringaldehyde, another bio-based building block, VS has been prepared via Wittig olefination (Rein et al., 2005), Knoevenagel–Doebner (Sinha et al., 2007), or Knoevenagel condensation-decarboxylation methods (van Schijndel et al., 2020).

4.2 Engineering a sinapic acid decarboxylase

In 2010, Matte and coworkers published the crystal structure of the PAD from *Bacillus pumilus* UI-670 (2010). Structural analysis of the PAD dimer revealed one monomer in an "open" conformation and the other monomer in a "closed" conformation, due to the differences in the conformation of a Asn15 residue on a flexible β1–β2 loop. Leading from the surface of the enzyme to the catalytic residues at the bottom of the cavity was a tunnel lined with several hydrophobic and hydrophilic residues including Ile21, Ile29, Ile33, Val38, Trp62, Thr66, Thr68, Val70, Leu72, Gly83, Ile85, Val91, and Thr98. The bottom of the cavity was closed off to solvent, suggesting the substrate and product would need to enter and leave through the same opening. Substrate specificity studies showed that the wild-type PAD enzyme from *Bacillus pumilus* UI-670 was able to decarboxylate FA, CA, and p-CA, but was unable to decarboxylate sinapic acid. The residues in the activity site cavity were identified as potential candidates for protein engineering studies to alter the substrate specificity of the *B. pumilus* PAD enzyme for sinapic acid decarboxylation.

To accomplish this objective, Morley and coauthors adopted a semi-rational engineering approach to select amino acids in the active site for site-saturation mutagenesis (SSM) (Morley et al., 2013). Efforts to co-crystallize PAD with ferulic acid or p-coumaric acid were unsuccessful, however a modeled PAD-FA complex structure was obtained by substrate docking and MD simulations. Using this model, five residues located within ~5 Å of the docked substrate were targeted for site-saturation mutagenesis: Tyr19, Val38, Val70, Ile85, and Phe87 (Figure 4.8). The site-saturation mutagenesis libraries were constructed by employing NNK codon degeneracy using the cloned PAD–encoding gene from *B. pumilus* UI-670 as a template.

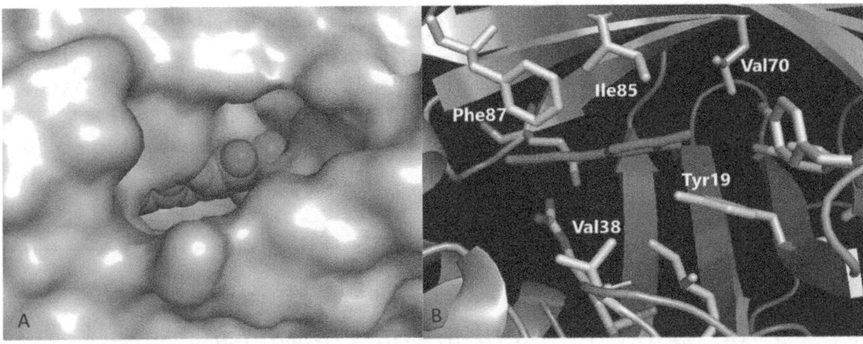

Figure 4.8 *B. pumilus* PAD active site model with FA. (A) Surface view of the open active site form of *B. pumilus* PAD. FA is shown in red. (B) Side-chain of the active site residues are labelled and shown as stick models. Ferulic acid is shown as a stick model in red (Morley et al., 2013).

The *Escherichia coli* transformants harboring the mutant libraries were grown on LB agar plates containing antibiotic. Approximately 192 colonies from each library were selected and recultured into 96-well plates for the subsequent activity screening assay. Enzymatic decarboxylation was monitored spectrophotometrically by measuring the decrease in SA absorbance at 310 nm over time. Of the five libraries, only the Ile85 library afforded hits with SAD activity. These hits were identified by DNA sequencing to be Ile85Ala, Ile85Gly, Ile85Ser, and Ile85Thr mutations of the enzyme. The four mutants were further analyzed using HPLC to evaluate their efficiency in the conversion of sinapic acid to 4-VS in 1-mL scale decarboxylation reactions. Ile85Ala (referred herein as SAD) afforded the highest amount of 4-VS and this enzyme was selected for protein purification and kinetic parameter determination.

The kinetic parameters were determined for wild-type PAD and SAD by the addition of different concentrations of substrates to the purified enzymes. For ferulic acid, the wild-type PAD and SAD had similar substrate affinities (K_m) of 2.7 and 3.2 mM, respectively (Table 4.1). However, the catalytic turnover (k_{cat}) was significantly decreased for SAD, resulting in a 6-fold reduction in the enzymes catalytic efficiency (k_{cat}/K_m) toward ferulic acid compared to wild-type PAD. There was no conversion of sinapic acid with wild-type PAD. For SAD, both the k_{cat} and K_m values were similar to those obtained with ferulic acid. Thus, a single amino acid replacement was found to expand the substrate specificity of PAD using a semi-rational approach.

Table 4.1 Kinetic parameters of wild-type PAD and SAD

Enzyme	substrate	Vmax (U mg^{-1})	K_m (mM)	k_{cat} (s^{-1})	k_{cat}/K_m ($s^{-1}M^{-1}$)
PAD	FA	273.1	2.7 ± 0.8	182 ± 20	6.7×10^4
SAD	FA	46.4	3.2 ± 0.3	31 ± 8	9.7×10^3
SAD	SA	41.3	3 ± 1	28 ± 4	9.3×10^3

Source: Morley et al. (2013).

4.3 *Process development for the enzymatic decarboxylation of SA and recovery of VS*

Various reaction solvents were explored in process development studies for the SAD–catalyzed decarboxylation of SA (Table 4.2). When the enzymatic decarboxylation of SA was performed in aqueous buffer, the concentration of SA was limited to ≤5 g/L due to product inhibition of the enzyme. Higher substrate concentrations or lower concentrations of the enzyme resulted in incomplete reactions (<95% conversion). Leisch and coworkers had previously demonstrated that wild-type PAD was inhibited by VG, the decarboxylation product of FA, even at low concentrations (0.25 g/L (Leisch et al., 2013). In this case, the addition of toluene as the immiscible organic solvent for in situ product removal, significantly improved the efficiency of the process.

The decarboxylation of SA with SAD was performed in biphasic reactions using either toluene, hexane, ethyl acetate, or the ionic liquid (BMIM)

Table 4.2 Decarboxylation of SA to VS in buffer and biphasic media

SA (g/L)	SAD (U/mL)[a]	Co-solvent[b]	% conv[c]	% isolated yield
5	10.6	None	95	75
25	2.0	None	37	30
25	2.0	Toluene	99	83
50	2.0	Toluene	50	45
50	4.0	Toluene	97	81
25	2	Ethyl acetate	42	n.d.[d]
25	2	Hexane	30	n.d.
25	2	$(BMIM)PF_6$	99.5	n.d.

Source: Morley et al. (2013).

[a] SAD was used as crude lysate.
[b] ratio of co-solvent to buffer was 1: 1 (v:v).
[c] determined by HPLC.
[d] n.d. = not determined.

PF_6 as a co-solvent. For the decarboxylation of 25 g/L SA, both biphasic reactions using toluene and (BMIM)PF_6 as co-solvents, proceeded to 99% conversion, whereas incomplete enzymatic reactions were observed using hexane and ethyl acetate. For the reaction using toluene, the product VS could be recovered in high purity by solvent extraction of the aqueous medium at acidic pH, and a slightly basic buffer wash of the combined organic extracts to remove the unreacted SA. In comparison, the recovery of VS from the ionic liquid by solvent extraction was not trival due to its high solubility in (BMIM)PF_6. Also, due to the high boiling point of the ionic liquid, VS could not be recovered by solvent evaporation. In summary, toluene was the best solvent to achieve both high reaction conversion and isolated yield of the product. By further optimizing the enzyme concentration in the decarboxylation reaction, up to 50 g/L of SA was converted to VS in the biphasic reaction.

4.4 Preparation of VS from canola meal extracts

For many years, canola meal has mainly been used as a high-protein source for animal feed. In addition to protein, canola meal is a source of phenolic compounds, including sinapic acid, sinapine, and sinapoyl glucoside (Wanasundara et al., 1994; Thiyam et al., 2006; Chen., 2016). To evaluate the potential of producing VS from canola meal extracts, a stepwise process combining chemical hydrolysis and enzymatic decarboxylation was explored by Morley et al. (2013). Alkaline treatment of 100 g of canola meal with sodium hydroxide extracted 780 mg of SA (7.8 mg/g). Initially, the SA was not recovered at this stage and an in situ enzymatic decarboxylation was performed on the neutralized canola meal extracts. However, the product VS was isolated in low purity due to contamination by residual fatty acids in the canola meal extracts. To overcome this issue, the purification procedure reported by Krygier et al. (1982) was followed for extracting free fatty acids and lipid components with hexane from canola meal extracts at acidic pH. The phenolic acids were then extracted with diethyl ether-ethyl acetate. The recovered SA was used without further purification in the biphasic decarboxylation with SAD. This reaction yielded 340 mg of VS in high purity (>90%), which corresponded to an overall yield of 3.0 mg VS/g of canola meal.

4.5 Polymerization of VS and characterization of PVS

Besides the interesting therapeutic properties of VS, this monomer serves as a building block for the biopolymer polyvinylsyringol (PVS). To evaluate the potential industrial applications of PVS, VS was polymerized under cationic conditions, as reported by Leisch et al. (2013), for the polymerization of VG to PVG. Treatment with boron trifluoride yielded a polymer

Table 4.3 Nanoindentation tests of PVS and PVG samples

Sample	Modulus, E (GPa)	Hardness, H (GPa)
PVS	5.22 ± 0.05	0.283 ± 0.003
PVG_{rad}	6.66 ± 0.05	0.421 ± 0.003
PVG_{cat}	6.75 ± 0.05	0.463 ± 0.006
PVG_{mixed}	6.5 ± 0.1	0.384 ± 0.012
PS 1301	4.15 ± 0.02	0.249 ± 0.001

Source: Morley et al. (2013).

with a number average molecular weight (Mn) of 10,764 and a polydispersity of 1.4. Thermal analysis of the PVS polymer by DSC revealed a glass transition temperature (T_g) range of 106°C–116°C, and a thermal stability of up to 350°C. In comparison, Nakamura et al. (1986) reported a T_g of 108°C for a PVS polymer obtained via hydrolysis of poly (4-acetoxy-3,5-dimethoxystyrene). The molecular weight (Mw) and polydispersity of this polymer were 9.9×10^4 and 3.7, respectively. In a more recent study by Takeshima et al. (2020), T_g values of 129°C and 110°C were determined for a PVS polymer and its silyl-protected hydroxy derivative.

Nanoindentation characterization of the produced PVS polymer, performed on polymer films compressed at 150°C following the CSM (continuous stiffness measurement), afforded hardness (H) and modulus (E) values that were slightly higher than the performance measured on commercial polystyrene PS 1301, which was analyzed simultaneously for comparison purposes (Table 4.3). On the contrary, the H and E values of PVS were significantly lower than the H and E values obtained for PVG polymers (Leisch et al., 2013). Based on these results, it is evident that altering the number and location of ring substituents can significantly influence the polymer properties.

4.6 *Recent advances in the development and application of sinapic acid decarboxylases*

Since the publication by Morley et al. (2013), there have been new reports of PADs exhibiting various levels of SAD activity. The PAD from *B. licheniformis* CGMCC 7172 (BLPAD) was reported to have a broader substrate specificity than previously characterized PADs (Hu et al., 2015). The recombinant BLPAD decarboxylated *p*-coumaric, ferulic, caffeic, and sinapic acids with specific activities of 157.96 ± 1.73, 117.82 ± 0.57, 54.36 ± 1.84, and 0.46 ± 0.02 Umg^{-1} (relative ratios of 100: 74: 34:0.3), respectively. In comparison, specific activities of 312 ± 40, 188 ± 2, 129 ± 4, and 1.0 ± 0.3 Umg^{-1} (relative ratios of 100:60:41:0.3) were reported for the wild-type *B. subtilis* PAD (Baraibar et al., 2016). However, in this study the enzyme activity toward sinapic acid was determined to be too low for scaling up the process. Low levels of SAD activity were also reported for the PAD from *Bacillus coagulans* DSM1. In this study, the PAD was co-expressed with an aromatic phenol monooxygenase to convert phenolic acids to aromatic aldehydes in a cascade process (Ni et al., 2018).

Schweiger and coworkers (2019) showed that mutation of the Ile85 residue in *B. subtilis* PAD improved its ability to decarboxylate sinapic acid, as observed for the *B. pumilus* PAD (van Schijndel et al., 2020). Ile85Ala, Ile85Val, and Ile85Leu mutants of BsPAD were generated by site-directed mutagenesis and tested for activity towards SA. Of the three mutants, Ile85Ala showed the highest decarboxylation activity with SA. In addition, this mutant was able to decarboxylate other sterically demanding substrates containing phenyl-ring substituents at the ortho and meta positions, whereas the wild-type PAD could not.

Another interesting application of the *B. pumilus* PAD Ile85Ala mutant involved its expression in developing seeds of *Camelina sativa* to reduce the sinapine content (Menard et al., 2022). Sinapine is considered an anti-nutritional in oilseed meal and one strategy for reducing its content is by modifying its biosynthetic pathway by genetic engineering (Figure 4.9). By introducing PAD activity into developing embryos of *C. sativa*, the hydroxycinnamic acid intermediates along the sinapine biosynthetic pathway were converted to their 4-vinyl derivatives, which resulted in a 95% reduction of sinapine content in the seeds. An increase in 4-VP and 4-VS content was detected in the engineered seeds, however the major metabolites were determined to be mono and diglycosylated derivatives of the vinylphenols.

A recent study by Li and coauthors aimed to improve the catalytic activity of the PAD from the *Bacillus amyloliquefaciens* ZJH-01 strain by engineering the N- and C-terminal region of the enzyme in combination with site-directed mutagenesis of active site residues (2021). In a rational design approach, they altered the sequence of *B. amyloliquefaciens* PAD to match the sequence of the N- and C-terminal regions and active site residues of a *Lactobacillus plantarum* PAD. For the wild-type enzyme, the specific activities were 13.44 ± 0.15, 3.16 ± 0.32, 2.87 ± 0.13, and 1.26 ± 0.06 Umg^{-1} (relative ratios of 100:24:21:9.4) for *p*-coumaric, ferulic, caffeic, and sinapic acid, respectively. The best improvement in specific activity (up to 4-fold increase) was obtained with a hybrid mutant containing the mutated N-terminal region and a His92Glu mutation in the active site.

Besides the methods reported for the production of VS using isolated PAD enzymes, the whole-cell bioconversion of SA into canolol by the filamentous fungi *Neolentinus lepideus* BRFM15 was also reported (Odinot et al., 2017). The strain was used in combination with an *Aspergillus niger* feruloyl esterase to hydrolyze sinapic acid from canola meal extracts and produce canolol in a two-step process. Concentrations up to 1.3 g/L of VS and 50 mg/L of syringic acid were reported for a 13-day cultivation study.

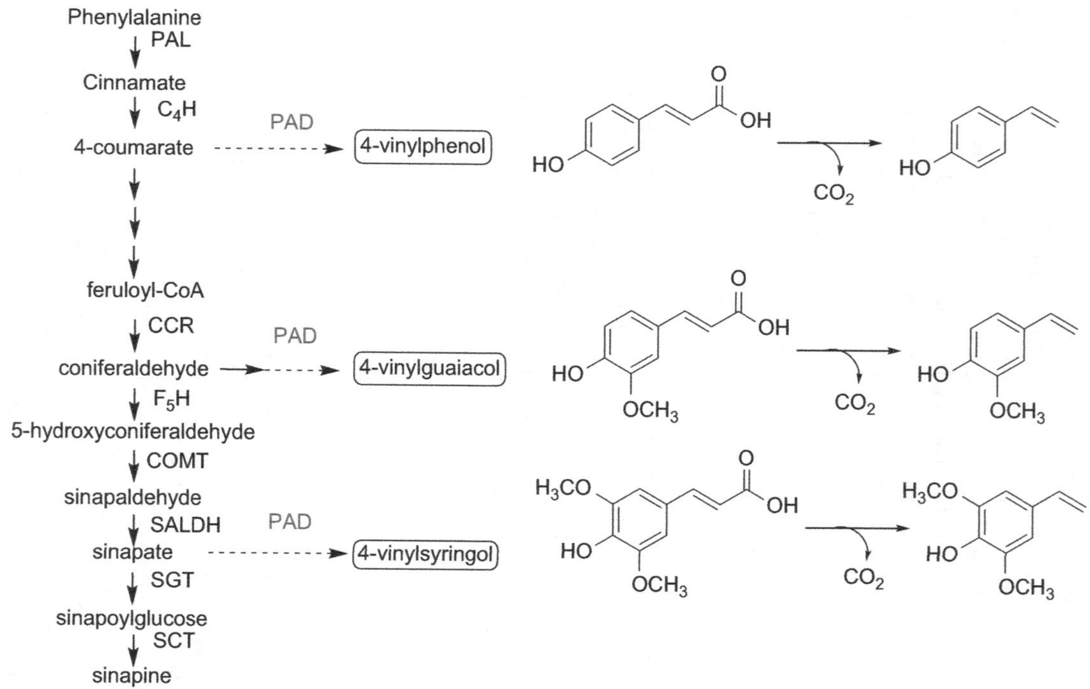

Figure 4.9 The main pathway of sinapoyl ester biosynthesis in Brassicaceous seeds.

(Diagram is adapted from Menard et al. (2022).

4.7 Conclusion

The chemoenzymatic route for converting canola meal to VS is just one example of using a naturally occurring or genetically modified enzyme to generate value-added products from a renewable feedstock. In addition to the production of value-added monomers like VS, the production of polyvinylphenols brings additional value to a biorefinery setting by expanding the portfolio of bio-based materials from the same bio-based feedstock. In bioprocess development, product recovery and purification are two essential parameters to consider when designing and optimizing an enzyme-catalyzed process. This chapter provided a brief overview of novel PADs identified with sinapic acid decarboxylase activity. Most technologies were in the early stages of development, thus the product VS had only been detected in the reaction media by analytical methods, and not extracted and fully characterized like the SAD–catalyzed process.

There has been significant progress over the last three decades in using protein engineering to improve the performance of enzymes as catalysts in synthetic organic chemistry and biotechnology. This chapter provided some insight into structure-based saturation mutagenesis, a semi-rational design strategy that uses information from enzyme crystal structures and in silico modeling to select amino acid positions for saturation mutagenesis. For the *B. pumilis* PAD, a single amino acid mutation in the active site was found to broaden the substrate specificity of PAD, while decreasing the catalytic efficiency of the enzyme. One strategy to further improve the catalytic properties of SAD could be iterative saturation mutagenesis, similar to the method that Reetz (2011) Wu et al. (2013) adopted to evolve both R- and S-selective mutants as catalysts for a variety of structurally different α-chiral esters. There has also been a lot of interest in utilizing biocatalysts in cascade processes to afford important building blocks for chemical synthesis. The combination of a sinapoyl esterase with SAD in a two-enzyme cascade process could potentially be a greener route for SA extraction from canola meal and transformation to VS.

References

Aachary, A. A., Chen, Y., Eskin, N. A. M., Thiyam-Hollander, U. (2014). Crude canolol and canola distillate extracts improve the stability of refined canola oil during deep-fat frying. *Eur. J. Lipid Sci. Technol.* 116, 1467–1476.

Abdelaziz, O. Y., Clemmensen, I., Meier, S., Costa, C. A. E., Rodrigues, A. E., Hulteberg, C. P., Riisager, A. (2022). On the oxidative valorization of lignin to high-value chemicals: A criticalrReview of opportunities and challenges. *ChemSusChem* 15, e202201232.

Baraibar, A. G., Reichert, D., Mügge, C., Seger, S., Gröger, H., Kourist, R. (2016). A one-pot cascade reaction combining an encapsulated decarboxylase with a metathesis catalyst for the synthesis of bio-based antioxidants. *Angew. Chem. Int. Ed.* 55, 14823–14827.

Barthelmebs, L., Diviès, C., Cavin, J. F. (2001). Expression in *Escherichia coli* of native and chimeric phenolic acid decarboxylases with modified enzymatic activities and method for screening recombinant E. coli strains expressing these enzymes. *Appl Environ Microbiol.* 67, 1063–1069.

Bernini, R., Mincione, E., Barontini, M., Provenzano, G., Setti, L. 2007. Obtaining 4-vinylphenols by decarboxylation of natural 4-hydroxycinnamic acids under microwave irradiation. *Tetrahedron* 63, 9663–9667.

Bourbiaux, D., Pu, J., Rataboul, F., Djakovitch, L., Geantet, C., Laurenti, D. (2021). Reductive or oxidative catalytic lignin depolymerization: An overview of recent advances. *Catalysis Today* 373, 24–37.

Cao, X., Tsukamoto, T., Seki, T., Tanaka, H., Morimura, S., Cao, L., Mizoshita, T., Ban, H., Toyoda, T., Maeda, H., Tatematsu, M. (2008). 4-Vinyl-2,6-dimethoxyphenol (canolol) suppresses oxidative stress and gastric carcinogenesis in *Helicobacter pylori*-infected carcinogen-treated Mongolian gerbils. *Int. J. Cancer* 122, 1445.

Cavin, J.-F., Barthelmebs, L., Guzzo, J., Van Beeumen, J., Samyn, B., Travers, J.-F. Diviès, C. (1997). Purification and characterization of an inducible p-coumaric acid decarboxylase from *Lactobacillus plantarum. FEMS Microbiol. Lett.* 147, 291–295.

Cavin, J.-F., Dartois, V., Divies, C. (1998). gene Cloning, transcriptional analysis, purification, and characterization of phenolic acid decarboxylase from *Bacillus subtilis. Appl. Environ. Microbiol.* 64, 1466–1471.

Chen, C. (2016). Sinapic Acid and Its derivatives as medicine in oxidative stress-induced diseases and aging. *Oxid. Med. Cell Longev.*, 2016, 10. Article ID 3571614, 2016.

Degrassi, G., Polverino De Laureto, P., Bruschi, C. V. (1995). Purification and characterization of ferulate and p-coumarate decarboxylase from Bacillus pumilus. *Appl Environ Microbiol.* 61, 326–332.

El-Seedi, H. R., El-Said, A. M. A., Khalifa, S. A. M., Göransson, U., Bohlin, L., Borg-Karlson, A.-K., Verpoorte, R. (2012). Biosynthesis, natural sources, dietary intake, pharmacokinetic properties, and biological activities of hydroxycinnamic Acids. *J. Agric. Food Chem.* 60, 10877–10895.

Faulds, C. B., Williamson, G. (1995). Release of ferulic acid from wheat bran by a ferulic acid esterase (FAE-III) from *Aspergillus niger. Appl Microbiol Biotechnol* 43, 1082–1087.

Fei Li, F., Zhao, Y., Xue, L., Ma, F., Dai, S. Y., Xie, S. (2022). Microbial lignin valorization through depolymerization to aromatics conversion. *Trends in Biotechnology* 40, 1469–1487.

Frank, A., Eborall, W., Hyde, R., Hart, S., Turkenburga, J. P., Grogan, G. (2012). Mutational analysis of phenolic acid decarboxylase from *Bacillus subtilis* (BsPAD), which converts bio-derived phenolic acids to styrene derivatives. *Catal. Sci. Technol.* 2, 1568–1574.

Gu, W., Yang, J., Lou, Z., Liang, L., Sun, Y., Huang, J., Li, X., Cao, Y., Meng, Z., Zhang, K.-Q. (2011). Structural basis of enzymatic activity for the ferulic acid decarboxylase (FADase) from Enterobacter sp. Px6-4. *PLOS ONE* 6, e16262.

Hashidoko, Y., Tahara, S. (1998). Stereochemically specific proton transfer in decarboxylation of 4-hydroxycinnamic acids by 4-hydroxycinnamate decarboxylase from Klebsiella oxytoca. *Arch Biochem Biophys.* 359, 225–230.

Hu, B., Zhang, Z.-X., Xie, W.-L., Liu, J., Li, Y., Zhang, W.-M., Fu, H., Lu, Q. (2022). Advances on the fast pyrolysis of biomass for the selective preparation of phenolic compounds. *Fuel Process. Technol.* 237, 107465.

Hu, H., Li, L., Ding, S. (2015). An organic solvent-tolerant phenolic acid decarboxylase from Bacillus licheniformis for the efficient bioconversion of hydroxycinnamic acids to vinyl phenol derivatives. *Appl. Microbiol. Biotechnol.* 99, 5071–5081.

Huang, Z., Dostal, L., Rosazza, J. P. (1993). Microbial transformations of ferulic acid by *Saccharomyces cerevisiae* and *Pseudomonas fluorescens*. *Appl. Environ. Microbiol.* 59, 2244–2250.

Huang, Z., Dostal, L., Rosazza, J. P. (1994). Purification and characterization of a ferulic acid decarboxylase from *Pseudomonas fluorescens*. *J. Bacteriol.* 176, 5912–5918.

Khattab, R., Eskin, M., Aliani, M., Thiyam, U. (2010). Determination of sinapic Acid derivatives in canola extracts using high-performance liquid chromatography. *J. Am. Oil. Chem. Soc.* 87, 147–155.

Krygier, K., Sosulski, F., Hogge, L. (1982). Free, esterified, and insoluble-bound phenolic acids. 1. Extraction and purification procedure. *J. Agric. Food Chem.* 30, 330–334.

Kumar, A., Jindal, M. Maharana, S., Thallada, B. (2021). Lignin biorefinery: New horizons in catalytic hydrodeoxygenation for the production of chemicals. *Energ. Fuels* 35, 16965–16994.

Kuwahara, H., Kanazaqa, A., Wakamatu, D., Morimura, S., Kida, K., Akaike, T., Maeda, H. (2004). Antioxidative and antimutagenic activities of 4-vinyl-2,6-dimethoxyphenol (canolol) isolated from canola oil. *J. Agric. Food Chem.* 52, 4380–4387.

Leisch, H., Grosse, S., Morley, K., Abokitse, K., Perrin, F., Denault, J., Lau, P. C. K. (2013). Chemicals from agricultural biomass: Chemoenzymatic approach for production of vinylphenols and polyvinylphenols from phenolic acids. *Green Process Synth.* 2, 7–17.

Li, Q., Xia, Y., Zhao, T., Gong, Y., Fang, S., Chen, M. (2021). Improving the catalytic characteristics of phenolic acid decarboxylase from *Bacillus amyloliquefaciens* by the engineering of N-terminus and C-terminus. *BMC Biotechnol.* 21, 44.

Matte, A., Grosse, S., Bergeron, H., Abokitse, K., Lau, P. C. K. (2010). Structural analysis of Bacillus pumilus phenolic acid decarboxylase, a lipocalin-fold enzyme. *Acta Cryst.* F66, 1407–1414.

Menard, G. N., Langdon, M., Bhunia, R. K., Shankhapal, A. R., Noleto-Dias, C., Lomax, C., Ward, J. L., Kurup, S., Eastmond, P. J. (2022). Diverting phenylpropanoid pathway flux from sinapine to produce industrially useful 4-vinyl derivatives of hydroxycinnamic acids in Brassicaceous oilseeds. *Metab. Eng.* 70, 196–205.

Morley, K. L., Grosse, S., Leisch, H., Lau, P. C. K. (2013). Antioxidant canolol production from a renewable feedstock via an engineered Decarboxylase. *Green Chem.* 15, 3312–3317.

Naczk, M., Amarowicz, R., Sullivan, A., Shahidi, F. (1998). Current research developments on polyphenolics of rapeseed/canola: A review. *Food Chem.* 62, 489–502.

Nakamura, K., Hatakeyama, T., Hatakeyama, H. (1986). DSC Studies on hydrogen bonding of poly(4-hydroxy-3,5-dimethoxystyrene) and related derivatives. *Polym J.* 18, 219–225.

Ni, J., Wu, Y.-T., Tao, F., Peng, Y. Xu, P. (2018). A coenzyme-free biocatalyst for the value-added utilization of lignin-derived aromatics. *J. Am. Chem. Soc.* 140, 16001–16005.

Nićiforović, N., Abramovič, H. (2014). Sinapic acid and its derivatives: Natural sources and bioactivity. *Compr. Rev. Food Sci. Food Saf.* 13, 34–51.

Odinot, E., Fine, F., Sigoillot, J.-C., Navarro, D., Laguna, O., Bisotto, A., Peyronnet, C., Ginies, C., Lecomte, J., Faulds, C. B. Lomascolo, A. (2017). A two-step bioconversion process for canolol production from rapeseed meal combining an *Aspergillus niger* feruloyl esterase and the fungus *Neolentinus lepideus. Microorganisms* 5, 67.

Pesci, L., Baydar, M., Glueck, S., Faber, K., Liese, A., Kara, S. (2017). Development and scaling-up of the fragrance compound 4-ethylguaiacol synthesis via a two-step chemo-enzymatic reaction sequence. *Org. Process Res. Dev.* 21, 85–93.

Reetz, M. T. (2011). Laboratory evolution of stereoselective enzymes: A prolific source of catalysts for asymmetric reactions. *Angew. Chemie.* 50, 138–174.

Rein, M. J., Ollilainen, V., Vahermo, M., Yli-Kauhaluoma, J., Heinonen, M. (2005). Identification of novel pyranoanthocyanins in berry juices. *Eur. Food Res. Technol.* 220, 239–244.

Rodríguez, H., Angulo, I., De Las Rivas, B., Campillo, N., Páez, J. A., Muñoz, R., Mancheño, J. M. (2010). *p*-Coumaric acid decarboxylase from *Lactobacillus plantarum*: Structural insights into the active site and decarboxylation catalytic mechanism. *Proteins* 78, 1662–1676.

Rosazza, J. P. N., Huang, Z., Dostal, L., Volm, T. Rousseau, B. (1995). Review: Biocatalytic transformation of ferulic acid, an abundant aromatic natural product. *J. Ind. Microbiol.* 15, 457–471.

Schweiger, A. K., Ríos-Lombardía, N., Winkler, C. K., Schmidt, S., Morís, F., Kroutil, W., González-Sabín, J., Kourist, R. (2019). Using deep eutectic solvents to overcome limited substrate solubility in the enzymatic decarboxylation of bio-based phenolic acids. *ACS Sustainable Chemistry and Engineering* 7, 16364–16370.

Sharma, A., Kumar, R., Sharma, N., Kumar, V., Sinha, A. K. (2008). Unique versatility of ionic liquids as clean decarboxylation catalyst cum solvent: A metal- and quinoline-free paradigm towards synthesis of indoles, styrenes, stilbenes and arene derivatives under microwave irradiation in aqueous conditions. *Adv. Synth. Catal.* 350, 2910–2920.

Sheng, X., Lind, M. E. S., Himo, F. (2015). Theoretical study of the reaction mechanism of phenolic acid decarboxylase. *FEBS J* 282, 4703–4713.

Sinha, A. K., Sharma, A., Joshi, B. P. (2007). One-pot two-step synthesis of 4-vinylphenols from 4-hydroxy substituted benzaldehydes under microwave irradiation: A new perspective on the classical Knoevenagel–Doebner reaction. *Tetrahedron* 63, 960–965.

Spielmeyer, A., Wagner, A., Jahreis, G. (2009). Influence of thermal treatment of rapeseed on the canolol content. *Food Chem.* 112, 944–948.

Sun, R., Sun, X. F., Wang, S. Q., Zhu, W., Wang, X. Y. (2002). Ester and ether linkages etween hydroxycinnamic acids and lignins from wheat, rice, rye, and barley straws, maize stems, and fast-growing poplar wood. *Ind. Crop. Prod.* 15, 179–188.

Takeshima, H., Satoh, K., Kamigaito, M. (2020). Bio-based vinylphenol family: Synthesis via decarboxylation of naturally occurring cinnamic acids and living radical polymerization for functionalized polystyrenes. *J. Polym. Sci.* 58, 91–100.

Terpinc, P., Polak, T., Segatin, N., Hanzlowsky, A., Ulrih, N. P., Abramovic, H. (2011). Antioxidant properties of 4-vinyl derivatives of hydroxycinnamic acids. *Food Chem.* 128, 62–69.

Thiyam, U., Stockmann, H., Felde, T. Z., Schwarz, K. (2006). Antioxidative effect of the main sinapic acid derivatives from rapeseed and mustard oil by-products. *Eur. J. Lipid Sci. Techol.* 108, 239–248.
van Schijndel, J., Molendijk, D., van Beurden, K., Canalle, L. A., Noël, T., Meuldijk, J. (2020). Preparation of bio-based styrene alternatives and their free radical polymerization. *Europ. Poly. J.* 125, 109534.
Wakamatsu, D., Morimura, S., Sawa, T., Kida, K., Nakai, C., Maeda, H. (2005). Isolation, identification, and structure of a potent alkyl-peroxyl radical scavenger in crude canola oil, canolol. *Biosci. Biotechnol. Biochem.* 69, 1568–1574.
Wanasundrara, U., Amarowicz, R., Shahidi, F. (1994). Isolation and Identification of an antioxidative component in canola meal. *J. Agric. Food Chem.* 42, 1285–1290.
Weiland, F., Kohlstedt, M., Wittmann, C. (2022). Guiding stars to the field of dreams: Metabolically engineered pathways and microbial platforms for a sustainable lignin-based industry. *Metab. Eng.* 71, 13–41.
Wu, Q., Soni, P., Reetz, M. T. (2013). Laboratory evolution of enantiocomplementary *Candida antarctica* Lipase B mutants with broad substrate scope. *J. Am. Chem. Soc.* 135, 1872–1881.
Yang, J., Wang, S., Lorrain, M.-J., Rho, D., Abokitse, K., Lau P. (2009). Bioproduction of lauryl lactone and 4-vinyl guaiacol as value-added chemicals in two-phase biotransformation systems. *Appl. Microb. Biotechnol.* 84, 867–876.
Yang, Q., Li, Y., Liu, H., Wang, E., Peng, M., Deng, T., Pan, X., Luo, Z., Yan, Y., Yang, L., Yang, X. (2022). Catalyst-free decarboxylation of 4-hydroxycinnamic acids: Efficient synthesis of 4-vinylphenols. *R. Soc. Open Sci.* 9, 220014.
Zago, A., Degrassi, G., Bruschi, C. V. (1995). Cloning, sequencing, and expression in *Escherichia coli* of the *Bacillus pumilus* gene for ferulic acid decarboxylase. *Appl. Environ. Microbiol.* 61, 4484–4486.
Zago, E., Dubreucq, E., Lecomte, J., Villeneuve, P., Fine, F., Fulcrand, H., Aouf, C. (2016). Synthesis of bio-based epoxy pre-polymers from natural ally- and vinyl phenols and the evaluation of their affinity to the endocrine receptor alpha by molecular docking. *New J. Chem.*, 40, 7701–7710.

chapter five

Antioxidant properties of canolol

Aleksander Siger, Krzysztof Dwiecki, and Ewa Bąkowska

5.1 Canolol – occurrence in vegetable oils

Canolol (2,6-dimetoxy-4-vinylphenol/ 4-vinylsyringol) is a derivative of sinapic acid (Figure 5.1). Seeds of rape and mustard (as well as other representatives of the genus *Brassica*) contain 10-fold greater amounts of phenolic compounds compared to other oil crops (Naczk and Shahidi 1992). They are particularly rich in sinapic acid and its derivatives. For this reason, canolol was for the first time identified in rapeseed oil in two independent studies by Koski et al. (2003) and Wakamatsu et al. (2005).

The primary factor contributing to the formation of this compound is connected with the application of elevated pressure and temperature in the process of oil extraction from seeds (Koski et al., 2003). Canolol content in raw rapeseed oil was 629 mg/kg, while in turnip oil it was 297 mg/kg (Koski et al., 2003). Siger et al. (2017b) compared contents of canolol in cold-pressed rapeseed oil (temperature of the matrix 60°C – temperature of oil 39°C) and hot-pressed oil (temperature of the matrix 90°C – temperature of oil 55°C). It was shown that raising the temperature of the matrix caused an increase in canolol contents in hot-pressed oil by 16%–20% compared to oil produced by cold pressing. Moisture content of seeds from which oil was pressed was another important parameter. Oils were pressed from seeds with moisture contents of 5%, 7.5%, and 10%.

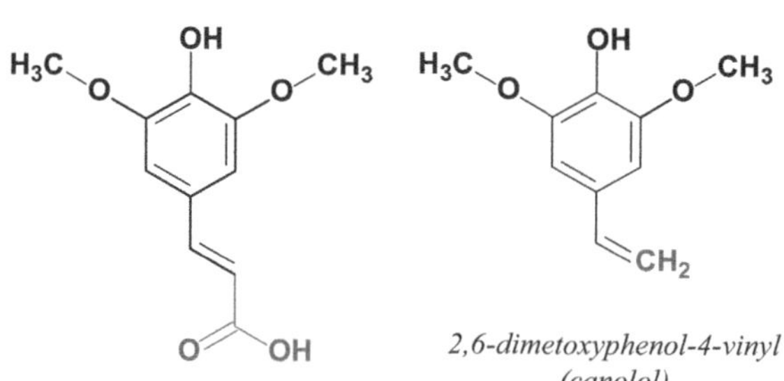

sinapic acid

2,6-dimetoxyphenol-4-vinyl (canolol)

Figure 5.1 Chemical structure of sinapic acid and its vinyl derivative – canolol.

DOI: 10.1201/b22828-5

The most optimal moisture content of seeds both in the case of cold and hot pressing was 7.5%. An increase in moisture contents of rapeseeds and the applied pressing method (cold pressing vs. hot pressing) had a significant effect on an increase in the contents of phenolic compounds in the tested oils. A greater effect was observed on the content of sinapic acid than on that of canolol. Contents of phenolic compounds, particularly sinapic acid, grew from 8.7 to 11.7 mg/kg and from 9.0 to 16.2 mg/kg, respectively, in cold-pressed vs. hot-pressed oils. It needs to be stressed that a 10% moisture content of rapeseeds highly significantly affected a decrease in oil yield, leading to poor pressing efficiency (Siger et al., 2016, 2017b). In other studies concerning cold-pressed oils from rapeseeds the content of canolol ranged from 5 to 140 mg/kg (Shrestha et al., 2012; Yang et al., 2014; Siger et al., 2015; Mildner-Szkudlarz et al., 2019). In degummed crude rapeseed oil its level was approx 200 mg/kg (Wakamatsu et al., 2005). Table 5.1 presents canolol content in vegetable oils. A marked increase in the level of canolol is observed in oils obtained from seeds subjected to heat treatment (convection or microwave heating), during which sinapic acid is decarboxylated, which finally leads to the formation of canolol. Wakamatsu et al. (2005) recorded from a 10- up to 100-fold increase in the content of canolol (549–1536 mg/kg) in rapeseed oils obtained from seeds roasted at a temperature of 160°C. Similar results were recorded for rape (Siger et al., 2015; Mildner-Szkudlarz et al., 2019) and mustard (Shrestha et al., 2012). Investigations conducted by Spielmeyer et al. (2009) were among the first studies illustrating a dependence between canolol contents in rapeseed oil and the applied microwave heating. Rapeseeds were exposed to the action of microwaves of 800 W for a period from 1.5 min up to 9 min, after which oil was extracted using petroleum ether. Based on the results, it was stated that canolol is a thermally unstable compound which is degraded at a temperature over 160°C (7 min, 800 W). According to the authors of this study, degradation of canolol at a high temperature is a result of its reaction with peroxide radicals formed when seeds are heated. The effect of microwave heating of rapeseeds on changes in canolol content in cold-pressed oil was presented by Yang et al. (2014). Heating of rapeseeds using microwave radiation of 800 W resulted in a reduction of canolol contents in oils pressed from seeds exposed to microwave radiation for 8 min. Different results are given by studies analyzing the effect of roasting of rapeseeds on canolol content in oil. Siger et al. (2015) recorded the highest content of canolol in oil pressed from seeds roasted for 15 min at a temperature of 180°C. In turn, Mayengbam et al. (2013) showed the highest increase in canolol level in oil pressed from seeds roasted for 15 min at 200°C. The application of the aforementioned parameters of heat treatment of seeds produced an over 2200-fold increase in the contents of canolol compared to oil extracted from unheated seeds.

Table 5.1 Canolol content in rapeseed oils subjected to preliminary heat treatment

Oils	Roasting conditions	Extraction method	Canolol (mg/kg)	References
Rapeseed (*Brassica napus*)	Unroasted	Cold pressing	177.12÷179.50	Siger et al. (2017b)
		Hot pressing	207.93÷216.67	
	Roasted (160°C/15 min)	Cold pressing	235.39÷263.59	
		Hot pressing	273.05÷285.00	
Yellow-seeded rapeseed (*Brassica napus*)	Unroasted	Cold pressing	8.53÷12.45	Siger et al. (2017a)
	Roasted (140°C/5–15 min)	Cold pressing	22.36÷132.28	
	Roasted (160°C/5–15 min)	Cold pressing	58.72÷258.93	
	Roasted (180°C/5–15 min)	Cold pressing	229.69÷768.26	
Rapeseed (*Brassica napus*)	Unroasted	Cold pressing	11.54	Siger et al. (2015)
	Roasted (140°C/5–15 min)	Cold pressing	29.36÷84.58	
	Roasted (160°C/5–15 min)	Cold pressing	121.40÷244.76	
	Roasted (180°C/5–15 min)	Cold pressing	328.98÷609.94	
Rapeseed (*Brassica napus*) Residual oil extracted from rapeseed expeller cake	Unroasted	Soxhlet extraction	24.56	Siger et al. (2016)
	Roasted (140°C/5–15 min)	Soxhlet extraction	71.93÷180.92	
	Roasted (160°C/5–15 min)	Soxhlet extraction	212.48÷413.67	
	Roasted (180°C/5–15 min)	Soxhlet extraction	98.40÷211.23	
Rapeseed (*Brassica napus*)	Microwave pretreatment (0 min)	Cold pressing	33.79	Rękas et al. (2018)
	Microwave pretreatment (2 min)	Cold pressing	39.18	
	Microwave pretreatment (4 min)	Cold pressing	60.94	
	Microwave pretreatment (6 min)	Cold pressing	286.96	
	Microwave pretreatment (8 min)	Cold pressing	895.35	
	Microwave pretreatment (10 min)	Cold pressing	1692.15	

Harbaum-Piayda et al. (2010) indicated potential formation of canolol dimers and trimers, which was confirmed in later studies, while two isomers of canolol dimers were also identified (*cis*- and *trans*- found at a 3:1 ratio) by Kraljić et al. (2015). Content of dimers in the deodistillate reaches 3500 mg/kg (Harbaum-Piayda et al., 2010).

5.2 *Antioxidant activity of canolol in homogeneous media*

The term "antioxidant" is widely used, but at the same time it is difficult to define precisely. Halliwell and Gutteridge (2015) proposed a broad definition of antioxidant as any substance found at a low concentration compared to the concentration of the oxidized substrate, which considerably delays or prevents oxidation of this substrate. In food technology antioxidants are to inhibit autoxidation of susceptible food components, including lipids, via several mechanisms of their action. Antioxidants may prevent initiation of lipid oxidation through chelation of metal ions or reduction of existing peroxides. Another potential mechanism consists in the inhibition of the free radical chain reaction through free radical scavenging. From the point of view of biology and nutrition, antioxidants may function in vivo to prevent oxidation of various biological targets and may include substances which chelate metal ions to prevent formation of reactive oxygen or nitrogen species (ROS or RNS); directly react with ROS or RNS and scavenge them; inhibit oxidative enzymes (e.g. lipoxygenases, cycloxygenases); or induce the activity of antioxidative enzymes.

Phenolic compounds belong to the group of most common antioxidants in our diet. At present a considerable role of polyphenolics has been confirmed in the prevention of cardiovascular diseases, cancers, and osteoporosis, while their prophylactic action has been suggested in the case of neurodegenerative diseases and diabetes (Espín et al., 2007). Studies are being conducted to clarify the mechanisms of action of phenolic compounds, while antioxidative properties are of major importance in the case of these compounds. For the phenolic compounds, which may be additives to enriched or functional food or components of dietary supplements, it is necessary to exercise particular caution when determining their dosage, considering for example the structure-activity dependence, bioavailability, metabolism, and antioxidant activity. Literature on the subject presents data on the occurrence of decarboxylation of hydroxycinnamic acids to 4-vinyl derivatives by intestinal bacteria (Nićiforović and Abramovič, 2014). In view of the preceding it may be assumed that microbial decarboxylation of sinapic acid in the colon may lead to the formation of canolol in the human organism, which means that this fact has to be taken into consideration when determining a safe dose for humans either as a component of functional food or a medication. Studies concerning contents and antioxidant activity of phenolic compounds (including sinapic acid and its derivatives) found, for example, in seeds of plants from the family *Brassicaceae*, have been conducted since the 1980s (Sosulski and Zadernowski, 1981; Naczk and Shahidi 1992; Vuorela et al., 2003; Kuwahara et al., 2004; Siger et al., 2013; Thiyam-Holländer et al., 2014; Wang et al., 2021). Antioxidant capacity of phenolic compounds is typically determined using several simple and rapid tests of antioxidant activity in vitro. Depending on the mechanism of the reaction these methods may be divided into those based on the hydrogen atom transfer (HAT) and single electron transfer (SET). In 2006, the sequential proton loss electron transfer (SPLET) mechanism was proposed by Zhang and Ji (2006). Methods based on the HAT mechanism include the oxygen radical absorbing capacity (ORAC) assay, total peroxyl radical trapping antioxidant potential (TRAP) test, crocin bleaching assay (CBA), and lipid peroxidation inhibition capacity (LPIC). In turn, methods based on the SET mechanism include the 2,2-diphenyl-1-picrylhydrazyl (DPPH) radical scavenging capacity assay, ABTS cation radical ($ABTS^{\bullet+}$) scavenging capacity assay, total phenolic contents assay using the Folin–Ciocalteu reagent (FCR), cupric ion reducing antioxidant capacity (CUPRAC), and the ferric ion reducing antioxidant parameter (FRAP).Some other methods are, for example,the superoxide anion radical ($O_2^{\bullet-}$) scavenging capacity assay, hydroxyl radical ($^{\bullet}OH$) scavenging capacity (HOSC), or total oxyradical scavenging capacity (TOSC) test. The SET and HAT reactions combined with the proton exchange reactions may be run simultaneously with the primary reactions and in such a case the dominant mechanism in a given system depends on the structure and properties of the antioxidant, solubility, and the distribution coefficient, as well as the solvent system (Munteanu and Apetrei, 2021). For this reason, antioxidant activity determined using various tests may show considerable discrepancies, thus simultaneous use of more than one antioxidant test is recommended in order to obtain more reliable results (Frankel and Meyer, 2000). Factors affecting antioxidant properties of phenolic compounds include contents of hydroxy groups and their location within the molecule, polarity, solubility, reduction potential, pH of the medium and dissociation constants of acids and bases (pKa) for the analyzed compounds, stability of phenols during technological processes, and stability of phenolic radicals (Pokorny, 2003; Akoh, 2008). Introduction of additional hydroxy groups to the aromatic ring enhances antioxidant activity. This results from the stabilization of phenoxyl radicals through the formation of a hydrogen bond between these groups. This leads to a greater activity of caffeic acid compared to that of coumaric acid. In turn, substitution of hydrogen in the hydroxy group with the methylene group (e.g. ferulic acid) has a varied effect on antioxidant properties depending on the polarity of the medium

(Rice-Evans et al., 1996). Derivatives of cinnamic acid exhibit greater antioxidant activity when compared to derivatives of benzoic acid. The higher antioxidant activity is caused by the presence of the -CH=CH-COOH group, which provides a greater capacity to release H and stabilize radicals than the -COOH group in hydroxybenzoic acids were of an opinion that the number of potential resonance structures of the phenoxyl radical results in the greater activity of cinnamic acid derivatives (Balasundram et al., 2006; Zhou et al. 2006).

One of the most popular methods used to assess the antioxidant capacity of food or extracts of phenolic compounds is the DPPH radical scavenging test. Canolol due to its strong fat solubility has proved to have good antioxidant properties (Yang et al., 2014). Koski et al. (2003) observed the antioxidant action of canolol and found that its protective activity in relation to lipids is similar to that of α-tocopherol. In turn, Kuwahara et al. (2004) stated that canolol, to a considerable extent, in a dose-dependent manner, reduces the intracellular apoptosis caused by oxidative stress. Those authors also showed that canolol prevents DNA strand disruption caused by $ONOO^-$. Wakamatsu et al. (2005) proposed that CNL is a more effective scavenger of alkyl peroxy radicals than α-tocopherol, vitamin C, β-carotene, rutin, or quercetin. This compound is also attributed for antimutagenic, anticancer, cytoprotective, and anti-inflammatory actions (Vuorela et al., 2003; Kuwahara et al., 2004; Wakamatsu et al., 2005; Galano et al., 2011a; Sørensen et al., 2013; Aachary et al., 2014). Galano et al. (2011a) investigated in detail the reaction of canolol with peroxide radicals. Its action, as a free radical scavenger, was investigated in aqueous and lipid solutions, while in the latter medium the reaction was 3.6-fold faster. It was found that the HAT mechanism, that is, hydrogen atom transfer from the phenolic radical of canolol, is the primary mechanism of this reaction and it was responsible for reactivity of this compound in relation to $^{\bullet}OOH$, which exceeded 99% regardless of the polarity of the medium. In a study by Vuorela et al. (2005) the antioxidant activity of the canolol standard in relation to DPPH radicals was lower than that of the sinapic acid standard. Canolol at a concentration of 0.5 and 1.0 mg/mL scavenged 37.1% and 78.7% DPPH radicals, respectively, while the values for the same concentration of sinapic acid amounted to 47.6% and 90.8%. However, the highest levels of scavenged DPPH radicals were recorded for the methanol extract of phenolic compounds obtained from rapeseed oil amounting to 65.4% (for the concentration of 0.5 mg/mL) and 93.8% (for the concentration of 1.0 mg/mL). This extract contained 87% canolol and 13% jointly sinapic acid and sinapin, which suggests the synergistic interaction between various phenolic compounds contained in rape seeds. This was confirmed by a study of Harbaum-Piayda et al. (2010) who showed that the antioxidant activity of extracts obtained from rapeseed oils in relation to DPPH (mM Trolox /kg oil) to a considerable extent depends on the total concentration (in mg/ kg) of phenolic compounds found in the extract. Terpinc et al. (2011) showed that the elimination of the carboxyl group in phenolic acids, except for *p*-coumaric acid, caused a considerable reduction (by over 50% compared to ferulic and sinapic acids and by 40% in the case of caffeic acid) of their DPPH radical scavenging capacity. Differences in the antioxidant activity between phenolic acids and products of their decarboxylation may be explained by their different structural characteristics, substitution in the aromatic ring, partition properties between lipids, and the aqueous phase as well as intermolecular interactions of hydrogen bonds.

Rękas et al. (2017a) investigated the effect of mechanical and thermal pretreatment of rapeseed on antioxidant capacity of oils with the DPPH radical, expressed in TEAC for total oil (TF) and for its hydrophilic (HF) and lipophilic fractions (LF). The radical scavenging activity (RSC) values in TF of oils pressed from hulled and unhulled seeds amounted to 1.52 and 1.65 mmol TEAC/L, respectively. The RSC value recorded for the lipophilic fraction of the control oils was higher than in the hydrophilic fraction, for oils obtained for hulled and unhulled seeds, respectively. It results from the preceding that the RSC of raw oils is mainly affected by the scavenging activity of lipophilic antioxidants, such as tocopherols and carotenoids. However, RSC of HF increased rapidly during thermal pretreatment of seeds. Specifically, the RSC value of HF increased 7- and 5-fold, respectively, after 10 min of microwave treatment and after 100-min roasting of hulled seeds. A respective increase in the antioxidant capacity of HF determined for oils pressed from hulled seeds was 8-fold to 6-fold. A considerable increase in RSC of HF results primarily from the thermally induced formation of canolol. A strong positive correlation between the concentration of canolol and RSC values of HF was recorded in oils pressed from microwaved seeds ($r = 0.941$) and roasted seeds ($r = 0.986$). A similar correlation was observed for oils pressed from hulled seeds, where Pearson's correlation coefficient was $r = 0.960$, both for microwaved and roasted seeds. Storage stability of phenolic compounds in oils produced from rapeseed subjected to microwave treatment was higher than in the control oil, which was confirmed by the calculated half-life ($t_{1/2}$). The half-life ($t_{1/2}$) for phenolic compounds present in rapeseed oil increased with the extension of seed heating time. For example, $t_{1/2}$ for canolol in the control oil was 5.8 months^{-1}, while an almost 3-fold longer half-life of canolol (16.8 months^{-1}) was recorded in oil from seeds microwaved for 10 min (Rękas et al. 2017b, 2018).

Yu et al. (2020) investigated the effect of three pretreatment methods (roasting, microwave, and steam explosion pretreatment) on values of DPPH, FRAP, and oxidation induction time (OIT) of pressed rapeseed oil. Results indicate that all the three pretreatment processes considerably increased oxidative stability of rapeseed oil. This increase was more marked in the sample subjected to steam pretreatment. Thus, when the steam-explosion pressure reached 1.0 MPa, values of DPPH, FRAP, and OIT of the tested rapeseed oil sample amounted to 270.12 μmol/100 g, 305.12 μmol/100 g, and 14.58 h, respectively. Compared to the values recorded for the samples not subjected to pretreatment, DPPH, FRAP, and OIT of steam-explosion treated oil increased 15.35-, 13.84-, and 0.37-fold, probably due to the high contents of phenolic compounds, particularly canolol. Canolol content in rapeseed oil was the highest when steam-explosion pressure reached 1.0 MPa, increasing from 41.21 to 2168.69 mg/kg, which was equivalent to a 52.63-fold increase in relation to samples not subjected to heat treatment as well as 124.36% and 112.30% increase in relation to samples roasted at high temperature and microwave treatment. Cong et al. (2020) tested derivatives of sinapic acid in 39 rape cultivars, which were subjected to microwave pretreatment, and investigated their role in increasing the oxidative stability of rapeseed oils. They determined the mean content of sinapic acid derivatives in rapeseeds, including (ordered here from the highest to the lowest content) sinapine (SP), sinapoyl glucoside (SG), disinapoyl gentiobioside (DSG), quercetin-sinapoyl-di-hexose-pentose (QSDG), sinapoyl malate (SM), disinapoyl glucoside (DDSG), and sinapic acid (SA). Following microwave treatment, the content of canolol in rapeseeds increased from zero to 61.6–761 mg/kg, while that of sinapic acid derivatives decreased. The degradation rate of SG, DDSG, DSG, SM, SA, and sinapine was 59.1%, 40.2%, 33.7%, 27.4%, 14.4%, and 11.3%, respectively. No correlations were found between sinapine and canalol. However, SG, DSG, SM, and DDSG were considered canolol precursors. Moreover, a positive correlation was found between the induction period (IP) and canolol content. Cong et al. (2019) showed that the DPPH scavenging capacity of the hull, cotyledon, endosperm, and entire rapeseed are 642, 3813, 4128, and 3378 μmol TE/100 g sample, respectively. After microwave treatment, DPPH scavenging capacity of the hull, cotyledon, endosperm, and whole rapeseed are 902, 3716, 4177, and 3197 μmol TE/100 g sample. They ranked derivatives of sinapic acid from compounds with the highest to those with the lowest antioxidant activity. This ordering was as follows: sinapine (SP) > sinapic acid (SA) > sinapoylcholine thiocyanate-glucoside (STPG) > disinapoyl gentiobioside (DSGG) > quercetin-sinapoyl-di-hexosepentose (QSDG) > sinapoylmalic acid (SM) > sinapoyl-glucoside (SG) > canolol.

Nithya and Subramanian (2017) in various antioxidant activity tests showed that depending on its concentration, sinapic acid scavenges both DPPH and ABTS radicals. At a concentration of 100 μg/mL sinapic acid scavenged 82% DPPH radicals and 86.5% ABTS radicals. Its activity in relation to the superoxide anion radical ($O_2^{\bullet-}$) amounted to 88.6%, while in relation to the nitric oxide radical it was 78%. Abdulkadar and Pari (2011) stated that sinapic acid showed good scavenging activity toward superoxide anion radical ($O_2^{\bullet -}$), which is formed from molecular oxygen by the addition of an electron. They showed that sinapic acid at a concentration of 50 μM scavenges 35.52% formed $O_2^{\bullet -}$. Zou et al. (2002) reported that the inhibitory action of sinapic acid was relatively strong (IC50 17.98 μM) in the scavenging activity of $O_2^{\bullet -}$ compared to the typical antioxidant, Trolox (IC50 = 7.24 μM). In their study, Terpinc et al. (2011) stated that decarboxylation had no effect on the activity of sinapic acid in scavenging of superoxide radicals, since the difference between the activity of sinapic acid and canolol was not considerable. Results showed the following pattern of $O_2^{\bullet -}$ scavenging activity for decarboxylation products of different hydroxycinnamic acids: 4-vinylcatechol > 4-vinylsyringol (canolol) ≈ 4-vinylguaiacol > 4-vinylphenol.

The hydroxyl radical (•OH) is one of the most reactive oxidants in biological systems (Halliwell and Gutteridge, 2015). Sinapic acid and its derivatives exhibit the capacity to scavenge •OH radicals, and their activity is comparable to that of ascorbic acid (Zou et al., 2002; Takaya et al., 2003). Galano et al. (2011b) investigated the scavenging activity of hydroperoxyl radical (•OOH) by sinapic acid and canolol in aqueous and lipid solutions applying the theory of functional density. Based on the pKa values of the –COOH group (4.19–4.47), it was concluded that at physiological pH (7.4) sinapic acid mostly (99.9%) exists in the anionic form (such as a carboxylate) and therefore this form must be considered when estimating its antioxidant activity in aqueous solutions. In reality it was confirmed that the anion form of sinapic acid is more reactive in relation to oxygen radicals compared to the neutral form. Those authors showed that polarity of the medium increases its reactivity – sinapic acid reacts approximately 32.6-fold faster in the aqueous solution than in a nonpolar medium. In the case of canolol an opposite dependence was observed, as it was shown that it reacts approximately 3.6-fold faster in the lipid medium than in an aqueous solution. The main mechanism of •OOH scavenging by sinapic acid consists in the hydrogen atom transfer (HAT) from the –OH group regardless of polarity of the medium and the dominant form of the antioxidant (carboxylate, neutral). In turn, the reaction of sinapic acid with •OH, $^\bullet OCl_3$, and $^\bullet OOCl_3$ is possible through the SET mechanism at diffusion-controlled rates, rapidly followed by deprotonation. For this reason, it is expected that sinapic acid is an excellent scavenger of these reactive forms. Efficacy of sinapic acid as the scavenger of •OOH was assessed as much higher compared to that of melatonin or allicin, whereas it is approximately 10 times lower than that of carotenoids. In turn, in the case of canolol it is comparable to the activity of carotenes, higher than the activity of allicin and greatly exceeds that of melatonin. It was also found that the reaction of canolol with •OOH runs 10 times faster than the reaction of sinapic acid both in a polar and nonpolar medium (Galano et al., 2011a, 2011b). The scavenging capacity of hypochlorite (ClO^-) by hydroxycinnamic acids was investigated by Firuzi et al. (2010). They showed the following order of efficacy: caffeic acid > sinapic acid > chlorogenic acid > ferulic acid > *p*-coumaric acid. Sinapic acid strongly inhibited the formation of 3-nitrotyrosine in protein, and its action was more effective than that of ascorbic acid or α-tocopherol, which confirms its capacity to scavenge peroxynitrite ($ONOO^-$) (Niwa et al., 1999; Zou et al., 2002).

Also, the canolol dimer exhibits high potential as an antioxidant. Harbaum-Piayda et al. (2010) showed the presence of dimer and trimer in refined rapeseed oil and deodistillate. They stated that canolol dimer is characterized by a 2-fold greater antioxidant potential compared to monomer (of canolol). Antioxidant activity determined by the DPPH method was 0.6 and 1.2 mmol Trolox equivalents/kg for canolol and its dimer. In turn, the reducing power (TEAC) for the dimer and monomer amounted to 2.2 and 3.9 mmol Trolox equivalents/kg. In turn, Kraljić et al. (2019) assessed the antioxidant activity of canolol and its dimer using the ORAC test, which measures the scavenging activity against the physiologically important peroxy radical, known to play a role in lipid oxidation in food and in the human organism (the analysis is conducted at physiological pH and the temperature of 37°C). The antioxidant activity of canolol dimer (84.0193 μM TE/mg canolol dimer) was almost 5-fold higher than that of canolol (17.8427 μM TE/mg monomer). A higher antioxidant activity is attributed to the presence of a larger number of hydroxy groups in the canolol dimer (Oehlke et al., 2017). Kraljić et al. (2019) reported that the canolol dimer shows greater stability than its monomer during a 5-month storage, probably thanks to its phenylindane structure, which seems to equip the dimer with greater stability. Those authors stored ethanol extracts of raw and edible rapeseed oil for 5 months at three different temperatures: in a freezer at –20°C, in a fridge at 4°C, and at room temperature, which ranged from 20°C to 25°C. The canolol dimer showed much better stability during storage than the monomer at all the three tested temperatures. After 5 months of storage over 85% initial concentration of the dimer was retained in ethanol extracts irrespective of storage conditions. However, it is recommended to store dimer extracts in a freezer, because their losses at the temperature of –20°C were below 5%. For comparison, already 1 month of monomer extract storage in a fridge led to losses of over 15% canolol. In turn, at room temperature this reduction exceeded 50%. Results recorded after 5-month storage at –20°C showed canolol losses of approximately 22%. Storage of the extract at the temperature of 4°C caused losses of over 50% initial canolol concentration, while in the extracts stored at room temperature canolol was completely degraded (Kraljić et al., 2019).

5.3 Canolol and the stability of vegetable oils (storage and thermal processing)

Many published research papers stress a dependence between canolol contents and oxidative stability of rapeseed oil (Shrestha and De Meulenaer, 2014; Yang et al., 2014). Moreover, enrichment of high-oleic rapeseed oil in canolol slows down the formation of primary and secondary oxidation products during frying (Matthäus, 2006). Matthäus et al. (2014) showed a very strong effect of the canolol-enriched extract (200, 500, and 750 mg/kg) on thermal stability of high-oleic rapeseed oil during deep-frying. The most important parameters used to assess the quality of used oils, triacylglycerol di- and polymers as well as the total content of polar compounds were lower after 30 h of frying compared to the commonly used antioxidants, TBHQ and rosemary extract. This shows that reactions typical to oil degradation during frying are slowed down by the addition of canolol. At the same time, canolol also improves the stability of α- and γ-tocopherol in oil. Zhou et al. (2019) fried potatoes, tofu, and vegetables in rapeseed oil containing different levels of canolol (528.9 *vs.* 250.5 mg/kg). They showed that a high canolol content improves stability (lower peroxide values, anisidine values, and malondialdehyde levels) in the frying medium. At a higher concentration canolol was degraded more slowly and it contributed to lower losses of other compounds exhibiting antioxidant properties, including phenolic compounds, by 58.4% and 80.3%, respectively, in oil with a high and low content of canolol. The application of air-frying as a roasting method for oil seeds may be an effective pretreatment increasing canolol recovery. Such a method was proposed by Fadairo et al. (2021). They showed that temperature had a considerable effect on the amount of obtained canolol and other lipophilic derivatives of sinapic acid. Optimal air frying conditions facilitating maximization of canolol content are the temperature of 170°C and 180°C for 15 min. However, heat treatment at 180°C for 20 min reduced the amount of canolol, while simultaneously increasing total phenolic compounds (assayed using the Folin-Ciocialteu reagent). The decrease in canolol content was explained by its interaction with free radicals or by dimerization. Siger et al. (2015) showed a correlation between antioxidant activity (with the application of the DPPH test) and content of canolol in cold-pressed rapeseed oils. A significant effect of time and roasting temperature of rapeseeds on the antioxidant activity of cold-pressed oils was found. This effect was directly proportional and correlated with canolol contents in tested samples. Pearson's correlation coefficient was $r = 0.97$ ($p < 0.0001$). In turn, when analyzing contents of phenolic compounds in oils a negative correlation was shown between total contents of phenolic compounds and antioxidant activity ($r = -0.52$; $p < 0.0001$). However, despite the 50-fold increase in canolol contents in the tested oils only a 2-fold increase in antioxidant activity was recorded in the sample obtained from seeds roasted at 180°C for

15 min. It also needs to be remembered that the increase in antioxidant activity may also be influenced, for example by Maillard reaction products which exhibit antioxidant action, as confirmed in many model systems, as well as some food products containing lipids (Rufián-Henares and Morales, 2007; Amarowicz, 2009). Shrestha and De Meulenaer (2014) showed that phospholipids and browning reaction products such as the Maillard reaction products may also be responsible for better oxidative stability of mustard and rapeseed oils obtained from roasted seeds. In the case of cold pressing it is the yield of oil that is a problem, since pomace contains large amounts of residual oil, which content may be as high as 27% (Thacker and Petri, 2009). In a study by Siger et al. (2016), a detailed analysis of canolol contents in residual oil showed that during pressing of oil from seeds roasted at 180°C most of this compound passes to the oil during pressing (74%–77%). An opposite dependence was found for samples of seeds roasted at 140°C and 160°C, where most canolol was retained in pomace (the amount of canolol passing to cold-pressed oil did not exceed 40%). It was shown that within the applied temperatures and roasting times a given level of canolol per the total fat content in rapeseeds may be obtained by increasing roasting temperature or extending roasting time at a lower temperature. At the same time, cold-pressed oils produced from roasted seeds are characterized by an extended shelf life, reaching 12 months (except for the roasting variant at 140°C for 5 min). These oils only after a year of storage exceeded maximum admissible peroxide values specified by Codex Alimentarius. Oils from roasted seeds were characterized by a smaller reduction of antioxidant activity (DPPH) during storage, which is attributed to their contents of canolol. After 6 months and after 12 months of storage a statistically significant correlation was shown between antioxidant activity and canolol contents ($r = 0.98$; $p < 0.0001$) (Siger and Michalak, 2016).

Siger et al. (2017b) compared cold and hot pressing, showing that the greatest amounts of canolol in oil are retained when pressing oil from seeds with the 7.5% moisture content in the case of both unroasted and roasted seeds. Obviously, oil from roasted seeds (160°C, 15 min) contained greater amounts of canolol (263.59 and 285.00 mg/kg in cold-pressed and hot-pressed oil, respectively). A different regularity was observed in the case of antioxidant activity, since the highest activity was recorded at the highest seed moisture content. This was caused by the higher contents of the other phenolic compounds in tested oils. In the case of hot pressing of oil from unroasted seeds the total content of phenolic compounds in oil increased from 9.0 mg/kg (for seeds with a 5% moisture content) to 12.5 mg/kg (for seeds with a 7.5% moisture content) and up to 16.2 mg/kg (for seeds with a 10% moisture content). Similar dependencies were reported in other variants of this experiment. In those oils particularly high increases were recorded for the content of sinapic acid (Siger and Józefiak, 2016).

Mikołajczak et al. (2019) compared oxidative stability of rapeseed oil and flaxseed oil with an addition of 4-vinyl derivatives of sinapic and ferulic acids (80 mg/100 g oil) in the Rancimat test (110°C). Stability of rapeseed oil (expressed as induction period – IP) with the addition of canolol and 4-vinylguaiacol in relation to oil with no additives increased from 8.8 to 9.08 h and 10.8 h, respectively. In the case of flaxseed oil 4-vinylguaiacol (3.0 h) also proved to be more effective, as compared to 1.96 h for flaxseed oil and 2.0 h for flaxseed oil with canolol. Added vinyl derivatives of ferulic and sinapic acids were almost entirely consumed during the induction time of the accelerated oxidation test, which resulted in an approximately 80% and 95% decrease in canolol and 4-vinylguaiacol contents, respectively. However, their use increased the retention of intact forms of most of the determined compounds. The use of canolol preserved at least 81% of squalene, sterols, and carotenoids in both oils. Unfortunately, this compound favored the loss of tocopherols in rapeseed oil (mainly of α-tocopherol) and α-linolenic acid in flaxseed oil Mikołajczak et al. (2019). The addition of 80 mg 4-vinylguaiacol per 100 g oil increased IP of rapeseed, flaxseed, and olive oils by approximately 13%–50% in relation to control oils (pure oils). For comparison, the positive effect of canolol addition amounted to as little as 2%–5% (Tańska et al. 2018). Sinapic acid and canolol significantly improve oxidative stability of purified triacylglycerols (TAG) of rapeseed oil, which was shown by Oehlke et al. (2017). Obtained results confirm that these compounds may be recommended as natural additives to vegetable oils or other food products.

5.4 Antioxidant activity of canolol in different lipid systems (bulk oils, emulsions, oleogels, liposomes)

The activity of antioxidants in food and biological systems depends on many factors, including colloid properties of substrates, oxidation conditions and stages, as well as the position of antioxidants in various phases. When testing natural antioxidants in vitro it is thus necessary to consider the composition of the system, the type of oxidizing substrate, the method to accelerate oxidation, oxidation testing methods, and the method applied to quantify the activity of antioxidants. Efficacy of an antioxidant depends also on the heterogeneity and heterogeneous phases of the system; the type of the lipid substrate, including its physico-chemical status and the degree of unsaturation; the type of initiators, particularly transition metals; and other components and their possible interactions (Frankel and Meyer, 2000). Hence, it is important to distinguish in which lipid system the autoxidation takes place (bulk oils, emulsions, oleogels, liposomes). Different systems affect the progress of the oxidation process and the activity of antioxidants.

Oleogels are semisolid systems with entrapped liquid oil in a three-dimensional network of self-assembled microcrystalline particles having colloidal dimensions (organogelators) (Martins et al., 2016). The inhibition of lipid oxidation by the mustard seed extract containing canolol in the oleogel with beeswax and bulk oil did not differ statistically significantly. However, such a difference was observed in the case of standard antioxidants such as Trolox and butylated hydroxytoluene (BHT). This can be attributed to the interactions between the organogelator and extract constituents, or the standard antioxidants. The addition of beeswax to oleogel may improve or inhibit the dispersibility of synthetic antioxidants and mustard seed phenolics in the oil phase. It may also affect the position of the antioxidant compounds at the water/oil interface. This phenomenon might possibly involve chemical interactions leading to changes in the chemical functionality of the compounds (Martinović et al., 2020). The antioxidant activity of sinapic acid and its derivatives (including canolol) in different lipid model systems was investigated by Martinović et al. (2019b). In the oleogel-based system the authors noted an increase in the activity of less polar compounds (especially 4-vinylsyringol and butyl sinapate) as compared with bulk oil. They suggested possible interactions of the less polar components with the oil structuring agent in oleogel. In water suspension of liposomes, the highest antioxidant effect was recorded for alkyl sinapates and 4-vinylsyringol. This is attributed to the lipophilic nature of these molecules, thanks to which they are present almost exclusively in the lipid phase of liposomes. On the contrary, in bulk oil more lipophilic derivatives of sinapic acid had lower antioxidant activities (alkyl sinapates, 4-vinylsyringol). In the studies on the effect of sinapic acid and its derivatives on lipid membrane peroxidation it was shown that 4-vinylsyringol influences the main gel-to-liquid phase transition of phosphatidylcholine liposomes. It is believed that the interference in free-radical-induced membrane peroxidation and the penetration into lipid bilayers of an antioxidant are correlated (Martinović et al., 2019a). Studies on flavonoids and isoflavones indicated that these compounds could reduce the mobility of free radicals in the lipid bilayer. Therefore, membrane fluidity decreases results in the inhibition of lipid peroxidation due to the slowing of free radical reactions (Arora et al., 2000). Canolol is incorporated deeply into the lipid bilayer, where it decreases fluidity in the gel state of the lipid membranes, while in the liquid state this effect weakens. 4-vinylsyringol has a small topological polar surface area (TPSA) in comparison to sinapic acid and its esters (ethyl sinapate, propyl sinapate, butyl sinapate). Such a TPSA value promotes its deeper incorporation into the lipid bilayer. However, it can only form three H-bonds compared to five in sinapic acid esters. This weakens its bonding potential and thus the effect on membrane fluidity. On this basis it may also be explained why the canolol rigidifying effect diminishes with increasing temperature. This reduces the interactions between 4-vinylsyringol and lipid molecules. The theoretically calculated distribution of lipophilicity on the molecular surface is well correlated with the ability of phenolic compounds to inhibit lipid peroxidation. In this case, antioxidant activity is arranged in the following order: butyl sinapate > propyl sinapate > 4-vinylsyringol > ethyl sinapate (Martinović et al., 2019a).

The antioxidant activity of 4-vinylsyringol measured by the β-carotene bleaching test in emulsion differs from that recorded in a homogeneous polar medium measured by the reducing power, Folin–Ciocalteu assay, superoxide anion scavenging activity assay, and the DPPH test. According to the β-carotene bleaching test the antioxidant activity of canolol exceeded sinapic acids by 15%. Antioxidant activity in multiphase systems is influenced by several parameters. Partitioning of phenolic compounds between the lipid and aqueous phase, which depends on the polarity of compounds, plays an important role. The retention time of compounds in reversed-phase HPLC is governed by their polarity. Therefore, partition properties of phenolic compounds can be estimated through composition data of the mobile phase and retention time. On this basis it was concluded that the value for the chromatographic partition of 4-vinylsyringol was 0.40, while for sinapic acid it was 0.25. Hence it may be confirmed that the higher partition of 4-vinylsyringol into the apolar phase corresponds to higher antioxidant activity in comparison with sinapic acid. This observation is in line with octanol–water partition coefficients (logP) calculated for 4-vinyl derivatives and parent hydroxycinnamic acids. Additionally, specific interactions (via hydrogen bonds) were observed between phenolic acids and an emulsifier, Tween 20, that decreases scavenging of alkylperoxyl radicals. This may explain why phenolic acids in emulsion show a lower efficiency in the deactivation of alkylperoxyl radicals compared to products of their decarboxylation. The same phenomenon may explain why 4-vinylcatechol exhibits lower antioxidant activity in emulsion than 4-vinylsyringol, despite having more hydrogen-donating groups and higher activity in the DPPH assay and during superoxide anion radical scavenging. Simultaneously, 4-vinylguaiacol having one methoxy group exhibits higher activity against alkylperoxyl radicals in emulsion when compared to canolol. It can be expected that the presence of the second methoxy group in 4-vinylsyringol should additionally introduce the factor stabilizing phenoxyl radical, enhancing radical scavenging ability with respect to 4-vinylguaiacol. It can be observed here again that high affinity for the lipid phase increases antioxidant activity in the emulsion system (Terpinc et al. 2011). The results of a study by Tańska et al. (2018) confirmed the higher activity of 4-vinylguaiacol than 4-vinylsyringol in typical apolar matrices of natural oils. Sørensen et al. (2013) found that differences in the antioxidant activity of canolol, sinapine, whole canola extract, sinapic acid, and stripped canola oil in the oil-in-water emulsion come mainly from different chains attached to the phenolic rings, which results in different polarity and thereby different location in the emulsions. In this study the relative order of the antioxidant activities of sinapic acid derivatives in emulsion was as follows: canolol > sinapine > canola extract > sinapic acid.

5.5 The effects of association colloids on canolol antioxidant activity

The process of lipid oxidation is perceived mainly in the context of the mechanism of chemical reactions (formation of free radicals). However, we still need to consider the position of molecules participating in the autoxidation process, particularly at the nano-emulsion interphase (Budilarto and Kamal-Eldin, 2015). Oils are not homogeneous liquids, but due to the presence of trace amounts of water (200–300 mg/kg), which is the residue from seeds and/or the refining process, are considered to be water-in-oil nanoemulsions (Kittipongpittaya et al., 2016; Barouh et al., 2022). Apart from triacylglycerols (98%–99%) and a slight amount of water vegetable oils also contain a wide range of minor oil components such as free fatty acids, phospholipids, tocopherols, sterols, and mono- and diacylglycerols (Homma et al., 2015). They are amphiphilic compounds, capable of reducing surface tension and accumulating at the oil-water interphase. These compounds after exceeding the critical micelle concentration (CMC) undergo self-organization, spontaneously forming aggregates and producing association colloids, such as reverse micelles. They are structural opposites of the micelles found in the oil-in-water emulsions, since in the case of oil the polar heads of surface-active molecules are pointed toward the trace amounts of water, while the nonpolar tails target the oil phase (Xenakis et al. 2010; Villeneuve et al., 2021). The formation of association colloids formed at the oil–water interphase physically accelerates lipid autoxidation. At the oil–water interphase amphiphilic lipid hydroperoxides and water-soluble metal ions also accumulate, which when reacting with each other lead to the formation of high-energy free radicals, which increase the rate of lipid oxidation (Kittipongpittaya et al., 2014). The best method to inhibit autoxidation is through the addition of an antioxidant, with the effectiveness of their action also influenced by association colloids. According to the polar paradox theory, apolar antioxidants are more effective in polar matrices, such as oil-water emulsions, while polar antioxidants are more effective on apolar matrices, such as oils. This is connected with the position of polar antioxidants at the oil–water interphase, that is, their penetration to sites where autoxidation is most intensive (Porter, 1980, 1993; Chaiyasit et al., 2007). Unfortunately, refining of vegetable oils removes most polar antioxidants, primarily phenolic compounds. Canolol, which is formed during decarboxylation of sinapic acid, one of the main phenolic compounds found in rapeseeds, is more hydrophobic compared to sinapic acid, thus it is more fat-soluble and bioavailable (Zhang et al., 2017). The difference in hydrophobicity of both these compounds also affects the formation and structure of association colloids in oil, as well as the process of lipid autoxidation. Structural analyses were conducted by Rokosik et al. (2020a) based on stripped rapeseed oil, using fluorescence measurements and the NBD-PE probe (N-(7-nitrobenz-2-oxa-1,3-diazol-4-yl)-1,2-dihexadecanoyl-sn-glycero-3-phosphoethanolamine). This amphiphilic molecule also accumulates at the oil–water interphase, with the hydrophilic group responsible for fluorescence facing the water phase, which also facilitates the localization of antioxidants added in the tests within the formed micelles. The authors established that sinapic acid does not form reverse micelles, although it is embedded in the association colloids of DOPC (1,2-dioleoyl-sn-glycero-3-phosphocholine) and it is found in their hydrophilic region. This is indicated, among other things, by the decrease in the fluorescence intensity of the stationary probe together with the increase in the concentration of sinapic acid in the presence of DOPC micelles. The interaction of sinapic acid with DOPC association colloids is also confirmed by the analysis of fluorescence anisotropy, where the reduction of anisotropy is observed at the increase in the concentration of sinapic acid in the presence of DOPC micelles. Analysis of anisotropy showed that sinapic acid, by embedding in the DOPC association colloids, changes their structure, which was observed in the increased rotational freedom of the NBD-PE probe. In turn, when measuring both stationary fluorescence and fluorescence anisotropy in oil samples together with an increase in the concentration of sinapic acid (without DOPC micelles), no statistically significant changes were observed, which suggests that sinapic acid alone does not form association colloids. Other evidence for the interaction of sinapic acid with DOPC association colloids was obtained using the method determining the fluorescence lifetime of the probe (Rokosik et al., 2020a). Based on the Stern-Volmer equation characterizing fluorescence quenching of the probe in the presence of sinapic acid, the value of the quenching constant was calculated, which informs whether dynamic quenching occurred in the oil ($kq<10^{10}$ $M^{-1}s^{-1}$) as a result of molecule collision or whether it was static quenching ($kq>10^{10}$ $M^{-1}s^{-1}$) due to the formation of a complex of the molecules (Czubinski et al., 2014). Obtained results ($kq = 2,5*10^{11}$ $M^{-1}s^{-1}$) by an order of magnitude higher than the boundary value confirm the formation of the NBD-PE probe complex (found in DOPC micelles) with sinapic acid and thus constitute further evidence for sinapic acid being embedded in the structure of association colloids (Rokosik et al., 2020a). In contrast, in the case of canolol other interactions occur for association colloids. This was confirmed by a study of Rokosik et al. (2020b), who used fluorescence measurements both to determine changes in fluorescence intensity and fluorescence anisotropy of the NBD-PE probe, as well as changes in the emission of fluorescence of canolol alone. Based on the recorded fluorescence of canolol in the presence and absence of DOPC, statistically significant differences may be observed between the emission of fluorescence in the control and at a high concentration of canolol (500 µmol/kg oil). This phenomenon may be explained by the change in the micromatrix of the antioxidant molecules, which suggests that canolol was embedded into the structure of DOPC association colloids. Additionally, fluorescence of the stationary NBD-PE probe was measured in samples of oil with canolol in the presence of DOPC in order to determine the position of canolol in DOPC micelles. No statistically significant changes were observed in the intensity of fluorescence emission of the NBD-PE probe, regardless of the canolol concentration in the presence of DOPC. This shows that canolol is not found in the hydrophilic part of the DOPC micelles, but it has the ability to interact with the hydrophobic area of the DOPC association colloids. However, the authors stressed that in contrast to sinapic acid, canolol is capable of forming association colloids, as indicated by the decrease in the fluorescence intensity of the stationary probe (a change in the environment) as well as the increase in fluorescence anisotropy of the probe (change of rotational freedom) in the oil together with the increasing concentration of canolol (Rokosik et al., 2020b). Rokosik et al. (2020b) also investigated the synergy between canolol and one of the main antioxidants found in rapeseed oil, that is, α-tocopherol. Structural analyses (measurement of stationary fluorescence using the NBD-PE probe) indicated that a mixture of canolol and α-tocopherol at high concentration of both antioxidants (each added at 500 µmol/kg oil) leads to changes in the hydrophilic region of DOPC association colloids, while mixtures of antioxidants alone at the investigated concentration (0–500 µmol/kg oil) do not form reverse micelles (Rokosik et al., 2020b).

Additionally, a team headed by Rokosik et al. (2020a, 2020b) also investigated autoxidation (the accelerated oxidation test at 55°C for 15 days) of stripped rapeseed oil with an addition of canolol and sinapic acid in the presence and absence of DOPC association colloids. It was confirmed that DOPC association colloids exhibit pro-oxidative action, which was also confirmed by Chen et al. (2011) in their studies on stripped soybean oil with an addition of DOPC (Chen et al., 2011; Rokosik et al., 2020a, 2020b). The addition of sinapic acid and canolol to oil had no effect on the formation of primary lipid oxidation products. In turn, in the case of secondary oxidation products (hexanal) the aforementioned antioxidants delayed the phase of hexanal formation; however, DOPC association colloids resulted in a reduced antioxidant efficiency of these antioxidants. Those authors also reported several differences in the antioxidant properties of sinapic acid and canolol despite similarities in their structure

(Rokosik et al., 2020a, 2020b). The efficacy of the antioxidant activity of canolol and sinapic acid was influenced by DOPC association colloids as well as by the concentrations of added antioxidants. In the case of sinapic acid, for the first 10 days the effect of primarily DOPC reverse micelles was observed. The sample of oil with an addition of sinapic acid at 10 μmol/kg oil was characterized by the slowest increase in hexanal content throughout the experiment. However, already the addition of DOPC (500 μmol/kg oil) to the aforementioned sample caused an increased rate of hexanal formation, which after 15 days of oxidation was almost 2-fold higher than in the oil sample with 10 μmol/kg oil sinapic acid (without DOPC) (Rokosik et al., 2020a). In turn, in the case of canolol the oil sample with the addition of a low concentration (10 μmol/kg oil) of this antioxidant in the presence of DOPC association colloids was already on the second day of oxidation characterized by pro-oxidative action, which was maintained until the 4th day. However, throughout the rest of the experiment the content of hexanal was comparable, while at day 15 in this sample (oil with an addition of DOPC and 10 μmol/kg oil canolol) the content of hexanal decreased by approximately 39% compared to the oil sample with DOPC. In turn, the sample of oil with DOPC and 100 μmol/kg oil canolol exhibited antioxidant action; however, toward the end of the experiment this action was completely inhibited (Rokosik et al., 2020b). Additionally, an increase in the concentration of oxidation products (lipid hydroperoxides and aldehydes), which due to their amphiphilic character will accumulate at the oil-water interphase (i.e. at the site of formation of association colloids), leads to increased oxidation rate through modification of micelle structures (Rokosik et al., 2020a, 2020b; Bąkowska et al., 2022).

Similar model studies based on the accelerated oxidation test (60°C for 20 days) were conducted on stripped soybean oil with an addition of sinapic acid, canolol, and α-tocopherol; however, no effect of association colloids was determined for the oil autoxidation process. Conducted studies showed that the most effective antioxidant was canolol (at 500 μmol/kg oil), which exhibited the highest antioxidant stability and the best capacity to inhibit degradation of linoleic and linolenic acids during the oxidation test (Wang et al., 2014). In turn, Oehlke et al. (2017) controlled the rate of formation of lipid hydroperoxides in stripped rapeseed oil with an addition of selected antioxidants (at a concentration of 200 μmol/kg oil), oxidized in the dark at a temperature of 40°C for 35 days. Those authors stated that the applied antioxidants markedly delayed the rate of lipid hydroperoxide formation and their antioxidant activity decreased in the following order: Trolox > canolol > synapic acid > BHA > tocopherol > canolol dimer. In this case the effect of antioxidants on stripped oil was also determined excluding the participation of association colloids Oehlke et al. (2017).

Phospholipids are components of both crude and refined oils and they form association colloids, most often in combination with other amphiphilic minor oil components. Phospholipids present in bulk oils include, among others, phosphatidylcholine (lecithin). It was found that the presence of phenolic compounds in rapeseed lecithin (canolol, sinapic acid) increases its antioxidant and ion-chelating capacities, probably due to the synergism between phenols and phospholipids (Robert et al., 2020). Oehlke et al. (2017) investigated antioxidant activity of deodorizer distillate fractions in rapeseed oil. The authors added fractions containing high amounts of vinylsyringol dimer (VSD) to commercial refined rapeseed oil. This increased the total VSD concentration in the oil from 13.5 to 42.3 mg/kg and resulted in a 2.5- to 3-fold slowdown in lipid oxidation. The authors attributed the observed effect to the presence of colloidal structures in the oil, such as reverse micelles.

Mikołajczak et al. (2022) noted that low antioxidant efficiency of canolol and guaiacol was recorded in cold-pressed oils from evening primrose and poppy seed having low initial quality, probably related to the presence of amphiphilic lipid autoxidation products (hydroperoxides, aldehydes, ketones, and others). These compounds form association colloids in bulk oil containing small amounts of water. The formed structures may, in turn, affect the oxidation process and diminish the antioxidant effectiveness of phenolic compounds. The effect of reverse micelles on the oxidation process of cold-pressed rapeseed and flaxseed oils in the presence of canolol was also highlighted in another paper (Mikołajczak et al., 2019).

A method to enhance antioxidant performance is also provided by their joint synergistic or additive action. Synergy is a phenomenon in which the activity of several compounds when they are found together in the same system is greater than the sum of their individual activities (Chaiyasit et al. 2007; Nogala-Kałucka et al., 2013). The best known example of such a synergistic action in the context of oils and heterogeneous lipid systems is the combination of vitamin E and vitamin C. Vitamin E inhibits the chain free radical reaction taking place during lipid oxidation, being transformed into the tocopherol radical, whereas vitamin C reduces its radical form to the original state, thus increasing the antioxidant efficacy of vitamin E (Packer et al., 2001). Literature also provides data on the interactions of canolol with other antioxidants. Rokosik et al. (2020a) determined mutual synergistic action of canolol and α-tocopherol in the presence and absence of DOPC association colloids in rapeseed oil. A synergistic action was observed for both these antioxidants after 15 days of the experiment (the accelerated oxidation test run at 55°C for 15 days) only in the presence of DOPC association colloids. Synergy of these antioxidants made it possible to eliminate the adverse effect of oxidation products on the efficacy of antioxidants. Additionally, the presence of canolol eliminated the pro-oxidative action of oil samples with an addition of DOPC and α-tocopherol, probably as a result of regeneration of α-tocopherol by canolol. Wang et al. (2014) investigated also the mutual antioxidant action of canolol and sinapic acid with α-tocopherol in stripped soybean oil. Those authors found no synergistic action in the case of these antioxidants; however, it needs to be remembered that the participation of association colloids was not investigated.

5.6 Conclusion

Vinyl derivatives of hydroxycinnamic acids, including the product of sinapic acid decarboxylation, canolol, have been extensively investigated in recent years. Canolol may be successfully applied as an antioxidant, which may be used outside of the food industry. Numerous studies showed the efficacy of canolol as an antioxidant in different lipid systems. Canolol, as a free radical scavenger, has been tested both in aqueous and lipid solutions. It was stated that the HAT mechanism, that is, hydrogen atom transfer from the phenolic group of canolol, is the main mechanism of this reaction and it is responsible for the antioxidant activity of this compound. It needs to be remembered that in the case of studies concerning antioxidant properties in vitro we need to consider the composition of the system, the type of the oxidized substrate, the method used to accelerate oxidation, and methods to assess oxidation as well as the method applied to quantify the activity of antioxidants. It is also necessary to take into consideration the position of molecules participating in the autoxidation process, particularly at the emulsion interphase. Due to the degradation of canolol during oxidation to dimer with documented antioxidant properties – as reported by some authors even exceeding those of the monomer itself – this compound proves to be an even more interesting object of study.

References

Aachary, A.A., Chen, Y., Eskin, N.A.M., Thiyam-Hollander, U. (2014). Crude canolol and canola distillate extracts improve the stability of refined canola oil during deep-fat frying: Deodistillates to stabilize frying oil. *Eur. J. Lipid Sci. Technol.* 116, 1467–1476.

Abdulkadar, M.J., Pari, L. (2011). Studies on the antioxidant and free radical-scavenging effect of sinapic acid: An *in vivo* and *in vitro* model. *J. Pharm. Sci. Res.* 3, 1447–1455.

Akoh, C.C. (2008). *Food Lipids Chemistry, Nutrition, and Biochemistry.* CRC Press/Taylor & Francis Group, Boca Raton, ISBN 978-1-4200-4554-9

Amarowicz, R. (2009). Antioxidant activity of Maillard reaction products. *Eur. J. Lipid Sci. Technol.* 111, 109–111.

Arora, A., Byrem, T.M., Nair, M.G., Strasburg, G.M. (2000). Modulation of liposomal membrane fluidity by flavonoids and isoflavonoids. *Arch. Biochem. Biophys.* 373, 102–109.

Bąkowska, E., Siger, A., Rudzińska, M., Dwiecki, K. (2022). Water content, critical micelle concentration of phospholipids and formation of association colloids as factors influencing autoxidation of rapeseed oil. *J. Sci. Food Agric.* 102, 488–495.

Balasundram, N., Sundram, K., Samman, S. (2006). Phenolic compounds in plants and agri-industrial by-products: Antioxidant activity, occurrence, and potential uses. *Food Chem.* 99, 191–203.

Barouh, N., Bourlieu-Lacanal, C., Figueroa-Espinoza, M.C., Durand, E., Villeneuve, P. (2022). Tocopherols as antioxidants in lipid-based systems: The combination of chemical and physicochemical interactions determines their efficiency. *Compr. Rev. Food Sci. Food Saf.* 21, 642–688.

Budilarto, E.S., Kamal-Eldin, A. (2015). The supramolecular chemistry of lipid oxidation and antioxidation in bulk oils. *Eur. J. Lipid Sci. Technol.* 117, 1095–1137.

Chaiyasit, W., Elias, R.J., McClements, D.J., Decker, E.A. (2007). Role of physical structures in bulk oils on lipid oxidation. *Crit. Rev. Food Sci. Nutr.* 47, 299–317.

Chen, B., Han, A., Laguerre, M., McClements, D.J., Decker, E.A. (2011). Role of reverse micelles on lipid oxidation in bulk oils: Impact of phospholipids on antioxidant activity of α-tocopherol and trolox. *Food Funct.* 2, 302.

Cong, Y., Cheong, L.-Z., Huang, F., Zheng, C., Wan, C., Zheng, M. (2019). Effects of microwave irradiation on the distribution of sinapic acid and its derivatives in rapeseed and the antioxidant evaluation. *LWT* 108, 310–318.

Cong, Y., Zheng, M., Huang, F., Liu, C., Zheng, C. (2020) Sinapic acid derivatives in microwave-pretreated rapeseeds and minor components in oils. *J. Food Compos. Anal.* 87, 103394.

Czubinski, J., Dwiecki, K., Siger, A., Neunert, G., Lampart-Szczapa, E. (2014). Characterisation of different digestion susceptibility of lupin seed globulins. *Food Chem.* 143, 418–426.

Espín, J.C., García-Conesa, M.T., Tomás-Barberán, F.A.2007. Nutraceuticals: Facts and fiction. *Phytochemistry.* 68, 2986–3008, doi:10.1016/j.phytochem.2007.09.014

Fadairo, O., Nandasiri, R., Alashi, A.M., Eskin, N.A.M., Thiyam-Höllander, U. (2021). Air frying pretreatment and the recovery of lipophilic sinapates from the oil fraction of mustard samples. *J. Food Sci.* 86, 3810–3823.

Firuzi, O., Giansanti, L., Vento, R., Seibert, C., Petrucci, R., Marrosu, G. Agostino, R., Saso, L. (2010). Hypochlorite scavenging activity of hydroxycinnamic acids evaluated by a rapid microplate method based on the measurement of chloramines. *J. Pharm. Pharmacol.* 55, 1021–1027.

Frankel, E.N., Meyer, A.S. (2000).The problems of using one-dimensional methods to evaluate multifunctional food and biological antioxidants. *J. Sci. Food Agric.* 80, 1925–1941.

Galano, A., Francisco-Márquez, M., Alvarez-Idaboy, J.R. (2011a). Canolol: A promising chemical agent against oxidative stress. *J. Phys. Chem. B* 115, 8590–8596.

Galano, A., Francisco-Márquez, M., Alvarez-Idaboy, J.R. (2011b). Mechanism and kinetics studies on the antioxidant activity of sinapic acid. *Phys. Chem. Chem. Phys.* 13, 11199.

Halliwell, B., Gutteridge, J.M.C. (2015). *Free Radicals in Biology and Medicine*, Fifth edition, Oxford University Press: Oxford, United Kingdom, ISBN 978-0-19-871747-8.

Harbaum-Piayda, B., Oehlke, K., Sönnichsen, F.D., Zacchi, P., Eggers, R., Schwarz, K. (2010). New polyphenolic compounds in commercial deodistillate and rapeseed oils. *Food Chem.* 123, 607–615.

Homma, R., Suzuki, K., Cui, L., McClements, D.J., Decker, E.A. (2015). Impact of association colloids on lipid oxidation in triacylglycerols and fatty acid ethyl esters. *J. Agric. Food Chem.* 63, 10161–10169.

Kittipongpittaya, K., Panya, A., Cui, L., McClements, D.J., Decker, E.A. (2014). Association colloids formed by multiple surface active minor components and their effect on lipid oxidation in bulk oil. *J. Am. Oil Chem. Soc.* 91, 1955–1965.

Kittipongpittaya, K., Panya, A., Decker, E.A. (2016). Role of water and selected minor components on association colloid formation and lipid oxidation in bulk oil. *J. Am. Oil Chem. Soc.* 93, 83–91.

Koski, A., Pekkarinen, S., Hopia, A., Wähälä, K., Heinonen, M. (2003). Processing of rapeseed oil: Effects on sinapic acid derivative content and oxidative stability. *Eur. Food Res. Technol.* 217, 110–114.

Kraljić, K. Brkan, V., Škevin, D., Srček, V.G., Radošević, K. (2019). Canolol dimer, a biologically active phenolic compound of edible rapeseed oil. *Lipids.* 54, 189–200.

Kraljić, K., Škevin, D., Barišić, L., Kovačević, M., Obranović, M., Jurčević, I. (2015). Changes in 4-vinylsyringol and other phenolics during rapeseed oil refining. *Food Chem.* 187, 236–242.

Kuwahara, H., Kanazawa, A., Wakamatu, D., Morimura, S., Kida, K., Akaike, T., Maeda, H. (2004). Antioxidative and antimutagenic activities of 4-vinyl-2,6-dimethoxyphenol (canolol) isolated from canola oil. *J. Agric. Food Chem.* 52, 4380–4387.

Martinović, N., Abramovič, H., Poklar Ulrih, N. (2019a). Inhibition of copper-induced lipid peroxidation by sinapic acid and its derivatives in correlation to their effect on the membrane structural properties. *Biochim. Biophys. Acta BBA - Biomembr.* 1861, 1–8.

Martinović, N., Poklar Ulrih, N., Abramovič, H. (2019b). Sinapic acid and its derivatives increase oxidative stability in different model lipid systems. *Eur. J. Lipid Sci. Technol.* 121, 1800326, doi:10.1002/ejlt.201800326

Martinović, N., Polak, T., Ulrih, N. P., Abramovič, H. (2020). Mustard seed: phenolic composition and effects on lipid oxidation in oil, oil-in-water emulsion and oleogel. *Ind. Crops Prod.* 156, 112851.

Martins, A.J., Cerqueira, M.A., Fasolin, L.H., Cunha, R.L., Vicente, A.A. (2016). Beeswax organogels: Influence of gelator concentration and oil type in the gelation process. *Food Res. Int.* 84, 170–179.

Matthäus, B. (2006). Utilization of high-oleic rapeseed oil for deep-fat frying of French fries compared to other commonly used edible oils. *Eur. J. Lipid Sci. Technol.* 108, 200–211.

Matthäus, B., Pudel, F., Chen, Y., Achary, A., Thiyam-Holländer, U. (2014). Impact of canolol-enriched extract from heat-treated canola meal to enhance oil quality parameters in deep-frying: A comparison with rosemary extract and TBHQ-fortified oil systems. *J. Am. Oil Chem. Soc.*, 91, 2065–2076.

Mayengbam, S., Khattab, R., Thiyam-Hollander, U. (2013). Effect of conventional and microwave toasting on sinapic acid derivatives and canolol content of canola. *Curr. Nutr. Food Sci.* 9, 321–327.

Mikołajczak, N., Tańska, M., Konopka, I. (2019). Impact of the addition of 4-vinyl-derivatives of ferulic and sinapic acids on retention of fatty acids and terpenoids in cold-pressed rapeseed and flaxseed oils during the induction period of oxidation. *Food Chem.* 278, 119–126.

Mikołajczak, N., Tańska, M., Ogrodowska, D., Czaplicki, S. (2022). Efficacy of canolol and guaiacol in the protection of cold-pressed oils being a dietary source of linoleic acid against oxidative deterioration. *Food Chem.* 393, 133390.

Mildner-Szkudlarz, S., Różańska, M., Siger, A., Kowalczewski, P.Ł., Rudzińska, M. (2019). Changes in chemical composition and oxidative stability of cold-pressed oils obtained from by-product roasted berry seeds. *LWT.* 111, 541–547.

Munteanu, I.G., Apetrei, C. (2021). Analytical methods used in determining antioxidant activity: A review. *Int. J. Mol. Sci.* 22, 3380.

Naczk, M., Shahidi, F. (1992). Phenolic constituents of rapeseed. In *Plant Polyphenols,* Hemingway, R.W., Laks, P.E., Eds., Springer US: Boston, MA. pp. 895–910 ISBN 978-1-4613-6540-2.

Nićiforović, N., Abramovič, H. (2014). Sinapic acid and its derivatives: Natural sources and bioactivity: Sinapic acid and its derivatives. *Compr. Rev. Food Sci. Food Saf.* 13, 34–51.

Nithya, R., Subramanian, S. (2017). Antioxidant properties of sinapic acid: In vitro and in vivo approach. *Asian J. Pharm. Clin. Res.* 2017, 10, 255.

Niwa, T., Doi, U., Kato, Y., Osawa, T. (1999). Inhibitory mechanism of sinapic acid against peroxynitrite-mediated tyrosine nitration of protein in vitro. *FEBS Lett.* 459, 43–46.

Nogala-Kałucka, M., Dwiecki, K., Siger, A., Górnaś, P., Polewski, K., Ciosek, S. (2013). Antioxidant synergism and antagonism between tocotrienols, quercetin and rutin in model system. *Acta Aliment.* 42, 360–370.

Oehlke, K., Harbaum-Piayda, B., Meyer, F., Eggers, R. Schwarz, K. (2017). Antioxidant Activity of Deodorizer Distillate Fractions in Rapeseed Oil. *Eur. J. Lipid Sci. Technol.*119, 1600273.

Packer, L., Weber, S.U., Rimbach, G. 2001. Molecular aspects of α-tocotrienol antioxidant action and cell signaling. *J. Nutr.* 131, 369S–373S.

Pokorny, J. (2003). *Antioxidants in Food: Practical Applications,* Woodhead publishing in food science and technology; Reprint., Woodhead: Cambridge. ISBN 978-0-8493-1222-9.

Porter, W.L. (1980). Recent trends in food applications of antioxidants. In *Autoxidation in Food and Biological Systems,* Simic, M.G., Karel, M., Eds., Springer US: Boston, MA, 1980, pp. 295–365 ISBN 978-1-4757-9353-6.

Porter, W.L. (1993). Paradoxical behavior of antioxidants in food and biological systems. *Toxicol. Ind. Health.* 9, 93–122.

Rękas, A., Ścibisz, I., Siger, A., Wroniak, M. (2017b).The effect of microwave pretreatment of seeds on the stability and degradation kinetics of phenolic compounds in rapeseed oil during long-term storage. *Food Chem.* 222, 43–52.

Rękas, A., Siger, A., Wroniak, M., Ścibisz, I. (2018). Phytochemicals and antioxidant activity degradation kinetics during long-term storage of rapeseed oil pressed from microwave-treated seeds. *Eur. J. Lipid Sci. Technol.* 120, 1700283.

Rękas, A., Wroniak, M., Siger, A., Ścibisz, I., Derewiaka, D., Anders, A. (2017a). Mechanical hulling and thermal pre-treatment effects on rapeseed oil antioxidant capacity and related lipophilic and hydrophilic bioactive compounds. *Int. J. Food Sci. Nutr.* 68, 788–799.

Rice-Evans, C.A., Miller, N.J., Paganga, G. (1996). Structure-antioxidant Activity relationships of flavonoids and phenolic acids. *Free Radic. Biol. Med.* 20, 933–956.

Robert, C., Couëdelo, L., Vaysse, C., Michalski, M.-C. (2020). Vegetable lecithins: A review of their compositional diversity, impact on lipid metabolism and potential in cardiometabolic disease prevention. *Biochimie.* 169, 121–132.

Rokosik, E., Siger, A., Rudzińska, M., Dwiecki, K. (2020b). Antioxidant activity and synergism of canolol and α-tocopherol in rapeseed oil is affected by the presence of phospholipid association colloids. *LWT.* 133, 110095.

Rokosik, E., Siger, A., Rudzińska, M., Siejak, P., Dwiecki, K. (2020a). Formation of phospholipid association colloids in rapeseed oil and their effect on lipid autoxidation in the presence of sinapic and ferulic acid. *Eur. J. Lipid Sci. Technol.* 122, 1900243.

Rufián-Henares, J.A., Morales, F.J. (2007). Functional properties of melanoidins: *In vitro* antioxidant, antimicrobial and antihypertensive activities. *Food Res. Int.* 40, 995–1002.

Shrestha, K., De Meulenaer, B. (2014). Effect of seed roasting on canolol, tocopherol, and phospholipid contents, Maillard type reactions, and oxidative stability of mustard and rapeseed oils. *J. Agric. Food Chem.* 62, 5412–5419.

Shrestha, K., Stevens, C.V., De Meulenaer, B. (2012). Isolation and identification of a potent radical scavenger (canolol) from roasted high erucic mustard seed oil from Nepal and its formation during roasting. *J. Agric. Food Chem.* 60, 7506–7512.

Siger, A., Czubinski, J., Dwiecki, K., Kachlicki, P., Nogala-Kalucka, M. (2013). Identification and antioxidant activity of sinapic acid derivatives in *Brassica napus* L. seed meal extracts. *Eur. J. Lipid Sci. Technol.* 115, 1130–1138.

Siger, A., Gawrysiak-Witulska, M., Bartkowiak-Broda, I. (2017a). Antioxidant (tocopherol and canolol) content in rapeseed oil obtained from roasted yellow-seeded *Brassica napus*. *J. Am. Oil Chem. Soc.* 94, 37–46, doi:10.1007/s11746-016-2921-7

Siger, A., Józefiak, M. (2016). The effects of roasting and seed moisture on the phenolic compoundlLevels in cold-pressed and hot-pressed rapeseed oil. *Eur. J. Lipid Sci. Technol.* 118, 1952–1958.

Siger, A., Józefiak, M., Górnas, P. (2017b). Cold-pressed and hot-pressed rapeseed oil: The effects of roasting and seed moisture on the antioxidant activity, canolol, and tocopherol level [Pdf]. *Acta Sci. Pol. Technol. Aliment.* 16, 69–81.

Siger, A., Kaczmarek, A., Rudzińska, M. (2015). Antioxidant activity and phytochemical content of cold-pressed rapeseed oil obtained from roasted seeds. *Eur. J. Lipid Sci. Technol.* 117, 1225–1237, doi:10.1002/ejlt.201400378

Siger, A., Michalak, M. (2016). The Long-term storage of cold-pressed oil from roasted rapeseed: Effects on antioxidant activity and levels of canolol and tocopherols. *Eur. J. Lipid Sci. Technol.* 118, 1030–1041.

Siger, A., Michalak, M., Rudzińska, M. (2016). Canolol, tocopherols, plastochromanol-8, and phytosterols content in residual oil extracted from rapeseed expeller cake obtained from roasted seed. *Eur. J. Lipid Sci. Technol.* 118, 1358–1367.

Sørensen, A.M., Friel, J., Winkler-Moser, J.K., Jacobsen, C., Huidrom, D., Reddy, N., Thiyam-Holländer, U. (2013). Impact of endogenous canola phenolics on the oxidative stability of oil-in-water emulsions. *Eur. J. Lipid Sci. Technol.* 115, 501–512.

Sosulski, F., Zadernowski, R. (1981). Fractionation of rapeseed meal into flour and hull components. *J. Am. Oil Chem. Soc.* 58, 96–98.

Spielmeyer, A., Wagner, A., Jahreis, G. (2009). Influence of thermal treatment of rapeseed on the canolol content. *Food Chem.* 112, 944–948.

Takaya, Y., Kondo, Y., Furukawa, T., Niwa, M. (2003). Antioxidant constituents of radish sprout (Kaiware-Daikon), *Raphanus sativus* L. *J. Agric. Food Chem.* 51, 8061–8066.

Tańska, M., Mikołajczak, N., Konopka, I. (2018). Comparison of the effect of sinapic and ferulic acids derivatives (4-vinylsyringol vs. 4-vinylguaiacol) as antioxidants of rapeseed, flaxseed, and extra virgin olive oils. *Food Chem.* 240, 679–685.

Terpinc, P., Polak, T., Šegatin, N., Hanzlowsky, A., Ulrih, N.P., Abramovič, H. (2011). Antioxidant properties of 4-vinyl derivatives of hydroxycinnamic acids. *Food Chem.* 128, 62–69.

Thacker, P.A., Petri, D. (2009). The effects of canola or mustard biodiesel press cake on nutrient digestibility and performance of broiler chickens. *Asian-Australas. J. Anim. Sci.* 22, 1531–1539.

Thiyam-Holländer, U., Aladedunye, F., Logan, A., Yang, H., Diehl, B.W.K. (2014). Identification and quantification of canolol and related sinapate precursors in Indian mustard oils and Canadian mustard products: Identification of canolol, sinapine and sinapic acid in mustard. *Eur. J. Lipid Sci. Technol.* 116, 1664–1674.

Villeneuve, P., Bourlieu-Lacanal, C., Durand, E., Lecomte, J., McClements, D.J., Decker, E.A. (2021). Lipid oxidation in emulsions and bulk oils: A review of the importance of micelles. *Crit. Rev. Food Sci. Nutr.* 63, 4687–47278.

Vuorela, S., Kreander, K., Karonen, M., Nieminen, R., Hämäläinen, M., Galkin, A., Laitinen, L., Salminen, J.-P., Moilanen, E., Pihlaja, K. (2005). Preclinical evaluation of rapeseed, raspberry, and pine bark phenolics for health related effects. *J. Agric. Food Chem. 53*, 5922–5931.

Vuorela, S., Meyer, A.S., Heinonen, M. (2003). Quantitative analysis of the main phenolics in rapeseed meal and oils processed differently using enzymatic hydrolysis and HPLC. *Eur. Food Res. Technol.* 217, 517–523.

Wakamatsu, D., Morimura, S., Sawa, T., Kida, K., Nakai, C. and Maeda H. (2005). Isolation. identification, and structure of a potent alkyl-peroxyl radical scavenger in crude canola oil, canolol. *Biosci. Biotechnol. Biochem.* 69, 1568–1574.

Wang, W., Yang, B., Li, W., Zhou, Q., Liu, C. Zheng, C. (2021). Effects of steam explosion pretreatment on the bioactive components and characteristics of rapeseed and rapeseed products. *LWT.* 143, 111172.

Wang, X.-Y., Yang, D., Zhang, H., Jia, C.-H., Shin, J.-A., Hong, S. T., Lee, Y.-H., Jang, Y.-S., & Lee, K.-T. (2014). Antioxidant activity of soybean oil containing 4-vinylsyringol obtained from decarboxylated sinapic acid. *JAOCS* 91, 1543–1550.

Xenakis, A., Papadimitriou, V. Sotiroudis, T.G. (2010). Colloidal structures in natural oils. *Curr. Opin. Colloid Interface Sci. 15*, 55–60.

Yang, M., Zheng, C., Zhou, Q., Liu, C., Li, W. Huang, F. (2014). Influence of microwaves treatment of rapeseed on phenolic compounds and canolol content. *J. Agric. Food Chem.* 62, 1956–1963.

Yu, G., Guo, T., Huang, Q. (2020). Preparation of rapeseed oil with superhigh canolol content and superior quality characteristics by steam explosion pretreatment technology. *Food Sci. Nutr. 8*, 2271–2278.

Zhang, H.-Y., Ji, H.-F. (2006). How vitamin E scavenges DPPH radicals in polar protic media. *New J. Chem.* 30, 503–504. https://pubs.rsc.org/en/content/articlelanding/2006/nj/b600025h

Zhang, J., Li, L., Wang, X., Wang, Z., Zheng, C., Zhang, H., Wang, H., Li, P., Zhai, X., Li, H., Tan, X. (2017). Inhibitory mechanism against oxidative stress and biological activities of canolol. *Acta Pol. Pharm. - Drug Res.* 74, 25–29.

Zhou, K., Yin, J., Yu, L. (2006). ESR Determination of the reactions between selected phenolic acids and free radicals or transition metals. *Food Chem.* 95, 446–457.

Zhou, Q., Jia, X., Deng, Q., Chen, H., Tang, H., Huang, F. (2019). Quality evaluation of rapeseed oil in Chinese traditional stir-frying. *Food Sci. Nutr.* 7, 3731–3741.

Zou, Y., Kim, A.R., Kim, J.E., Choi, J.S., Chung, H.Y. (2002). Peroxynitrite scavenging activity of sinapic acid (3,5-dimethoxy-4-hydroxycinnamic acid) isolated from *Brassica Juncea*. *J. Agric. Food Chem.* 50, 5884–5890.

chapter six

Anti-cancer properties of canolol

Xia Xiang and Zhenxia Xu

6.1 Introduction

Cancer is one of the greatest threats to human health and continues to be a global burden (Seyed et al., 2016). Approximately 90% of all cancers have an environmental cause, mainly through lifestyle (diet, smoking, outdoor pollution) while the remaining are due to genetics (Klaunig, 2018). Published literature suggested that oxidative stress and inflammation are closely linked to the initiation and progression of cancer. Canolol, an excellent orally bioavailable phenol from rapeseed oil, is a decarboxylated derivative of sinapic acid during the heat processing of rapeseed (Zhang et al., 2017). As a naturally potent antioxidant, canolol is far more effective at scavenging alkylperoxyl radicals than known antioxidants, like vitamin C, β-carotene, α-tocopherol, quercetin, and rutin (Kuwahara et al., 2004). Moreover, canolol can also suppress the production of nitric oxide synthase (iNOS) and inflammatory cytokines such as tumor necrosis factor-α (TNF-α), interleukin-1β (IL-1β), cyclooxygenase-2 (COX-2), and interferon-γ (IFN-γ) (Cao et al., 2008). According to these studies, canolol may act as a cancer chemopreventive and therapeutic agent by its antioxidant or anti-inflammatory effect.

6.2 Gastric cancer

Gastric cancer ranks fifth in incidence and is the third-leading cause of cancer-related death worldwide (Bray et al., 2018). There are several risk factors for this condition, including *Helicobacter pylori* infection, old age, alcohol use, high salt intake, and a diet low in fruits and vegetables (Smyth et al., 2020). *Helicobacter pylori* play an important role in gastric cancer development, which leads to chronic gastritis and peptic ulcer, and eventually gastric carcinoma (Den Hoed and Kuipers, 2016). Treatment includes surgery, perioperative or adjuvant chemotherapy, and sequential lines of chemotherapy.

Maeda et al. (2006) explored the inhibitory effect of canolol on bacterial mutagenesis and carcinogenesis in the *Helicobacter pylori*–infected gerbil model. Administration of canolol suppressed over 90% of mutation

DOI: 10.1201/b22828-6

caused by $ONOO^-$ exposure, inhibited the production of NO in mouse peritoneal macrophages model, and reduced IL-12 and TNF-α production. And mice with 0.1% canolol-enriched diet greatly suppressed the incidence of carcinoma formation in the stomach to about 35% of the control using a *Helicobacter pylori*–infected Mongolian gerbil model. Similarly, an investigation was also conducted using the above model to evaluate the effectiveness of canolol as an inhibitor for *Helicobacter pylori*–induced gastric carcinogenesis. It was found that dietary administration of 0.1% canolol markedly suppressed gastric carcinogenesis by inhibiting the mRNA expression of iNOS, COX-2, and inflammatory cytokines TNF-α, IL-12, and IL-1β, and alleviating serum 8-OHdG level and anti–*Helicobacter pylori* IgG titers caused by *Helicobacter pylori* infection, but not the inhibition of *Helicobacter pylori* colonization (Cao et al., 2008). Jiang et al. (2013) showed that canolol treatment inhibited cell proliferation in the human gastric cancer cell line (SGC-7901). In comparison with viable normal human gastric epithelial cells (GES-1), the inhibitory effect was dose-dependent. In addition, canolol-induced cell apoptosis through downregulating COX-2 mRNA expression level. To understand how canolol exerts its anticancer properties, Cao et al. (2015) demonstrated that the initiation and progression of gastric tumors in K19-C2mE transgenic (Tg) mice were suppressed when canolol was administered, which was done by blocking COX-2/PGE2 signaling pathway. These researchers discovered that treatment with canolol reduced the tumor incidence to 41.2% with a significant reduction in tumor size from 6.5 to 4.5 mm. In addition, canolol administration downregulated pro-inflammatory cytokine expression (COX-2, IL-1β, and IL-12b) and four key factors involved in PGE2 signal transduction (COX-2, EP2, Gαs, and β-catenin). In a recent study, the effects of canolol on human gastric carcinoma (AGS) cells were conducted (Han et al., 2019). It revealed that canolol inhibited the proliferation of AGS cells in a dose-dependent manner, manifested by decreased cell viability. Furthermore, canolol was shown to induce apoptosis of AGS cells by damaging mitochondrial membrane potential (MMP), increasing ROS level, arresting the cell cycle at the S phase, and mediating the abnormal protein expression of Bax, Bcl-2, caspase-3, and caspase-9 through PI3K/Akt signaling pathway (Figure 6.1).

6.3 *Cervical cancer*

Cervical cancer is the second most common gynecological malignancy globally, with high morbidity and mortality (He et al., 2021). Apoptosis reactivation has become the main strategy for inhibiting cancer proliferation (Montoya-Gómez et al., 2020). There is a need to extend the search for new potential drug candidates to implement less toxic and more effective

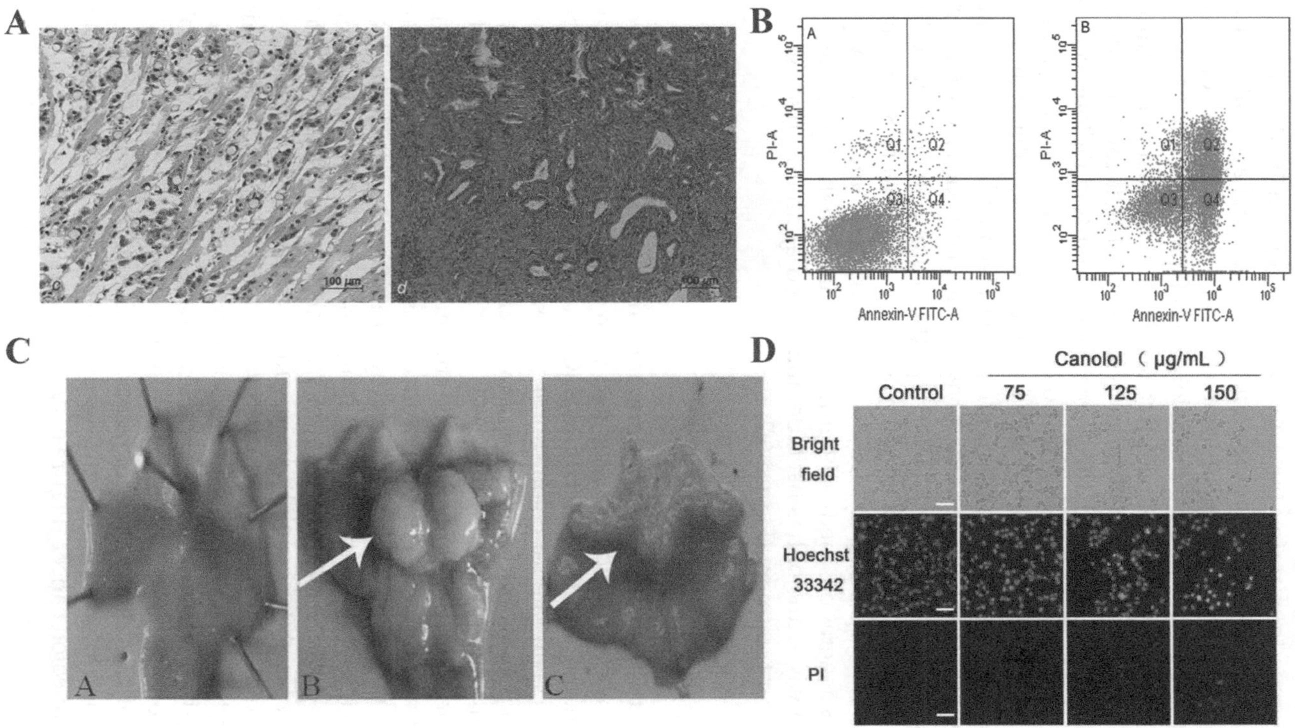

Figure 6.1 Histopathological features and histology characteristics of adenocarcinomas in gastric mucosa (A), apoptosis of SGC-7901 gastric cancer cells using flow cytometry (B), macroscopic images of gastric tissue in wild mice, Tg mice and canolol-treated Tg mice (C), and apoptosis induced by canolol in AGS cells using Hoechst 33342 and propidium iodide staining (D) (Cao et al., 2008; Jiang et al., 2013; Cao et al., 2015; Han et al., 2019).

strategies for cervical cancer treatment. Recently, Kraljić and coworkers used cytotoxicity-based CellTiter 96 AQueous one solution cell proliferation assays to examine the effects of canolol and its dimer on the proliferation of cervical adenocarcinoma cell line (HeLa) (Kraljić et al., 2019). Dose-dependent suppression of HeLa cell viability was observed with different concentrations of canolol (50–500 μM) for 72 h. Moreover, canolol exhibited lower cytotoxic effects on cell viability than its dimer. And results from flow cytometric analysis showed that canolol induced cell apoptosis and increased the percentage of early apoptotic cells to 13.25%. Xia et al. (2019) explored the potential of canolol for the treatment of cervical cancer. In vitro results showed that canolol exhibited anti-proliferative and apoptosis-promoting effects on HeLa cells with time- and dose-dependent manner, while demonstrating low toxicity on HEK-293 and LO2 cells. In vivo study of HeLa xenografts mouse model found that canolol significantly reduced tumor volume by 46.8% over 28 days, with tumor growth suppressed by 45.7%. Canolol triggers apoptosis by promoting ROS generation, mediating mitochondrial signaling pathway, and MAPK pathway. Canolol has been demonstrated as an effective agent in cervical cancer treatment (Figure 6.2).

6.4 Colon cancer

Colon cancer is one of the most commonly diagnosed digestive cancers, the development of which is associated with many factors, such as diet, microorganisms, and their metabolites (Chen and Shen, 2020). The overall 5-year survival rate for colon cancer patients is approximately 64% as a result of advances in treatment options such as colectomy, chemotherapy, and immunotherapy (Miller et al., 2019). Fang et al. (2013) studied the inhibitory effect of canolol on the inflammatory bowel disease and the development of colitis-related cancer based on an azoxymethane/dextran sulfate sodium-induced colon cancer mouse model. Through this investigation, about 40% of mice receiving canolol diet did not have colon tumors, compared with the control mice, which developed colon cancer in 100% of cases. After canolol administration, the number of tumors significantly reduced into 5.6±2.0 while that was 10.8 ± 4.2 in untreated mice. Meanwhile, the expression of inflammatory cytokines COX-2, TNF-α, and iNOS as well as HO-1 at the mRNA level were suppressed by canolol. They also found that colon 26 solid tumors were showed in decreased expression of COX-2 after canolol treatment. Despite this, canolol did not inhibit tumor growth significantly, so they concluded that it may potentially prevent colon cancer (Figure 6.3).

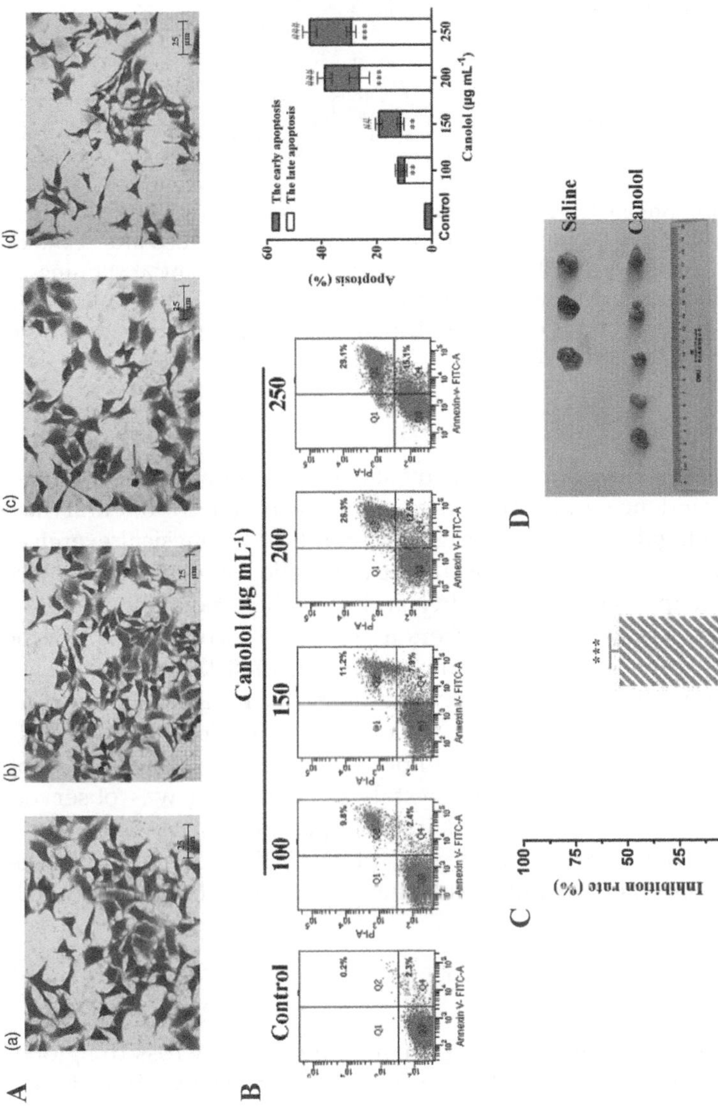

Figure 6.2 Optical microscopy of crystal-violet stained HeLa cells after 72 h pretreatment with different concentrations of canolol (A: control HeLa cells (a); cells treated with canolol 50 μM (b); 200 μM (c) and 500 μM (d)), the Annexin V-FITC/PI flow cytometry analysis of canolol-induced apoptosis in HeLa cells (B), the inhibition rate of canolol on HeLa xenografted tumors (C) and representative images of excised cervical cancer tumors from BALB/c nude mice on the 28th day (D) (Kraljić et al., 2019; Xia et al., 2019).

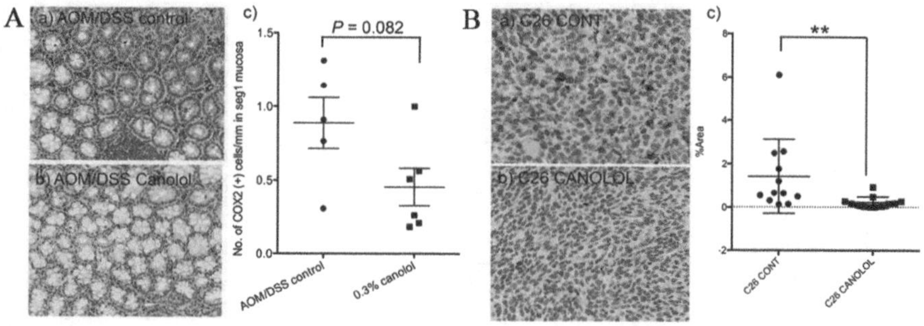

Figure 6.3 Inhibition of COX-2 expression in colonic tissue of AOM/DSS-treated ICR mice (A) and colon 26 transplanted tumor (B) in Balb/c mice after canolol administration. Panels A-a and B-a show the immunohistochemical staining of COX-2 in the control group tissues, A-b and B-b present the staining results in the canolol-treated groups, and A-c and B-c display the quantitative analysis of the COX-2–positive (brown) areas (Fang et al., 2013).

6.5 *Breast cancer*

In women, breast cancer remains the most common type of cancer. There is mounting evidence indicating the influence of environmental factors and lifestyle (alcohol intake, high-fat diet, lack of physical exercise) on breast carcinoma development, thereby nutrition and lifestyle interventions may help decrease morbidity and mortality (Kolak et al., 2017). In recent study, Kraljić and coworkers assessed in vitro cytotoxicity of canolol and its dimer as the anti-cancer agent against the MCF-7 breast adenocarcinoma cell line. They observed a decrease in MCF-7 cancer cells viability after treated by canolol at various concentrations (50–500 μM) for 72 h with the half maximal inhibitory concentration values (IC_{50}) of 318.25 μM. Cell morphology with crystal-violet staining was observed under light microscopy, and changes in the appearance of canolol-treated versus control cells were visible (Kraljić et al., 2019). Canolol possesses anti-breast cancer potential, but the mechanism needs to be further investigated (Figure 6.4).

6.6 *Liver cancer*

As the most common cause of cancer-related mortality across the globe, liver cancer is the only one of the top five lethal cancers with an annually increasing incidence (Siegel et al., 2019). The most frequent form of liver cancer is hepatocellular carcinoma that accounts for 80%–90% of all cases (Llovet et al., 2021). The well-established risk factors for the initiation

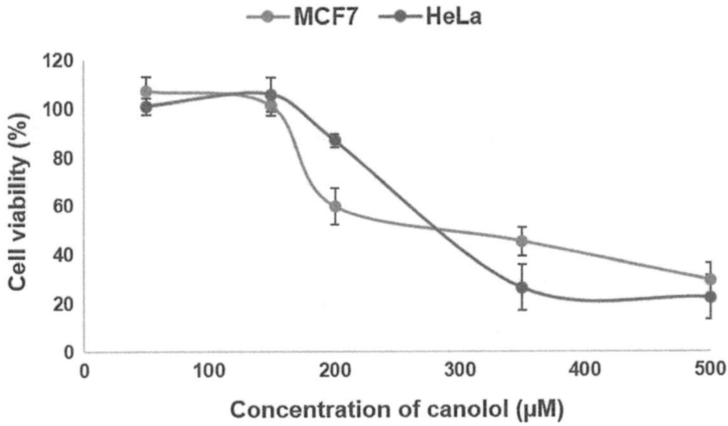

Figure 6.4 Effects of various concentrations of canolol on the viability of MCF7 and HeLa cells evaluated with the CellTiter 96 AQueous One Solution Cell Proliferation kit (Kraljić et al., 2019).

and development of liver cancer include chronic hepatitis B or hepatitis C virus infection, alcohol abuse, smoking, metabolic diseases such as non-alcoholic fatty liver disease, obesity and diabetes, and aflatoxin exposure (Yang et al., 2020). Xu et al. (2020) explored the effect of oven, infrared, and microwave pretreatment on rapeseed oil based on the contents and biofunctional activities of phenolic compounds. These researchers discovered that microwave pretreatment increased the phenolic compound contents, like sinapic acid and canolol, more than oven and infrared preprocessing in the oil. Furthermore, using Annexin V–FITC/PI staining, they investigated the impact of canolol on the apoptosis of HepG2 cells and found that low concentrations of canolol (10 and 100 μmol/L) displayed decent cell apoptotic inhibitory activity (23.06% and 16.94%), while the proportion of apoptotic cells after treatment with high concentrations of canolol (300 and 500 μmol/L) was slightly higher (33.73% and 35.53%). Canolol with low concentration increased Bcl-2 expression levels, upregulated the Bcl-2/Bax ratio, inhibited Bax, p53 and caspase-3 expression in HepG2 cells. Interestingly, low concentrations of canolol expressed its antiapoptotic effect through p53–Bax–Bcl-2–caspase-3, whereas the antiapoptotic activity of high concentrations of canolol were limited (Xu et al., 2020). Canolol, the main phenolic compound in rapeseed oil, exhibited appreciable antioxidant and antiapoptotic properties that are related to rapeseed oil quality (Figure 6.5).

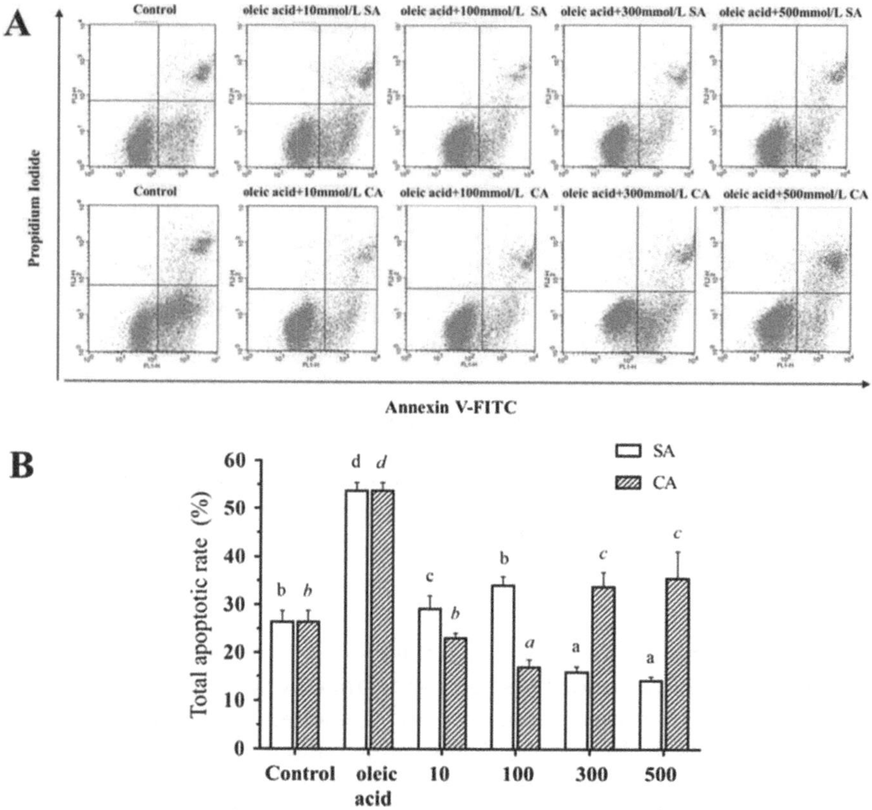

Figure 6.5 Effects of sinapic acid and canolol on oleic acid-induced apoptosis of HepG2 cells. Cell apoptosis of sinapic acid and canolol for 24 h treatment detected by using Annexin V–FITC/PI staining (A), and the total apoptotic rate of HepG2 cells treated with various concentrations of sinapic acid and canolol (B) (Xu et al., 2020).

6.7 Summary and conclusion

At present, dietary polyphenols are widely used for the treatment of many diseases, including metabolic disorders, autoimmune diseases, and cancer. Owing to the mild side effects and low cost, traditional therapy methods incorporating natural phenolic compounds, especially in cancer treatment, have garnered considerable attention from the global scientific and medical community. 4-vinyl-2,6-dimethoxyphenol named canolol, a phenolic compound isolated from crude rapeseed oil, exhibited potent anticancer and health-promoting properties. By adopting the in vitro cellular and in vivo preclinical animal models, the effects of canolol on regulating various types of cancers, such as gastric cancer, cervical cancer, colon cancer, breast cancer, and liver cancer, have been widely investigated in many previous studies. Canolol has been demonstrated to have beneficial effects against carcinogenesis and was considered as a natural promising anti-cancer agent. Studies showed that the anti-cancer effects of the canolol were multifaceted and complex, and the most reported possible mechanisms were attributed to their roles in stimulation autophagy and apoptosis of tumor cells, suppression of inflammatory response, modulation of cellular signaling cascades, and induction of oxide stress, epigenetic regulation, and inhibition of cell proliferation (Table 6.1). Yet it is worth noting that the anti-cancer activities of canolol were assessed only by animal and cell experiments in all these previous researches, thus, concerns have been raised that all these studies did not take into account the complexity of the in vivo metabolism of canolol. The stability and bioavailability of canolol were two major concerns. Therefore, more efforts are needed in this particular area to better understand the potential benefits of canolol for human health, and more clinic evidence, particularly human studies, is also necessary. With the development of deep studies in anticancer, canolol has a number of applications in the food, nutraceutical, and medical arenas.

Table 6.1 Canolol-treated cancer types, mechanisms, and relevant references

Cancer types	Mechanisms	References
Gastric cancer	Suppressed inflammatory cytokine production	Maeda et al. (2006)
	Decreased the mRNA expression of iNOS, COX-2 and pro-inflammatory cytokines TNF α,IL-12 and IL-1β Lowered serum 8-OHdG level	Cao et al. (2008)
	Down-regulated COX-2 mRNA expression	Jiang et al. (2013)
	Blocked COX-2/PGE2 signaling pathway	Cao et al. (2015)
	ROS generation, MMP damage, and cell-cycle arrest in the S phase Upregulated Bax expression, downregulated Bcl-2 expression, and activated caspase-9 and caspase-3 activity through PI3K/Akt signaling pathway	Han et al. (2019)
Cervical cancer	Inhibited cell growth and induced apoptosis	Kraljić et al. (2019)

(*Continued*)

Table 6.1 (Continued)

Cancer types	Mechanisms	References
	Induced oxidative stress Caused lysosomal membrane permeabilization Modulated mitochondrial signaling pathway by downregulating Bcl-2 expression and upregulating Bax, the ratio of Bax/Bcl-2, Cyt C, cleaved caspase-9, cleaved caspase-3 and cleaved-PARP Regulated MAPK pathway mediated with inactivation of the ERK1/2 and activation of the JNK and p38	Xia et al. (2019)
Colon cancer	Suppressed the expression of TNF-α, COX-2, iNOS and HO-1	Fang et al. (2013)
Breast cancer	Inhibited cell proliferation and induced apoptosis	Kraljić et al. (2019)
Liver cancer	Increased Bcl-2 expression levels Upregulated the Bcl-2/Bax ratio Inhibited Bax, p53 and caspase-3 expression levels Expressed its antiapoptotic activity through p53–Bax–Bcl-2–caspase-3	Xu et al. (2020)

References

Bray, F., Ferlay, J., Soerjomataram, I., Siegel, R., Torre, L., Jemal, A. (2018). Global cancer statistics 2018: GLOBOCAN estimates of incidence and mortality worldwide for 36 cancers in 185 countries. *CA: A Cancer Journal for Clinicians* 68, 394–424.

Cao, D., Jiang, J., Tsukamoto, T., Liu, R., Ma, L., Jia, Z., Kong, F., Oshima, M., Cao, X. (2015). Canolol inhibits gastric tumors initiation and progression through COX-2/PGE2 pathway in K19-C2mE transgenic mice. *PloS One* 10, e0120938.

Cao, X., Tsukamoto, T., Seki, T., Tanaka, H., Morimura, S., Cao, L., Mizoshita, T., Ban, H., Toyoda, T., Maeda, H., Tatematsu, M. (2008). 4-Vinyl-2,6-dimethoxyphenol (canolol) suppresses oxidative stress and gastric carcinogenesis in *Helicobacter pylori*-infected carcinogen-treated Mongolian gerbils. *International Journal of Cancer* 122, 1445–1454.

Chen, S., Shen, X. (2020). Long noncoding RNAs: functions and mechanisms in colon cancer. *Molecular Cancer* 19, 167.

den Hoed, C., Kuipers, E. (2016). Gastric cancer: How can we reduce the incidence of this disease? *Current Gastroenterology Reports* 18, 34.

Fang, J., Seki, T., Tsukamoto, T., Qin, H., Yin, H., Liao, L., Nakamura, H., Maeda, H. (2013). Protection from inflammatory bowel disease and colitis-associated carcinogenesis with 4-vinyl-2,6-dimethoxyphenol (canolol) involves suppression of oxidative stress and inflammatory cytokines. *Carcinogenesis* 34, 2833–2841.

Han, L., Xia, X., Deng, Q., Zheng, C., Zhang, Z., Ji, Q., Xiang, X. (2019). Canolol induces apoptosis in human gastric carcinoma cell through PI3K/Akt signaling pathway. *Oil Crop Science* 4, 244–253.

He, M., Xia, L., Li, J. (2021). Potential mechanisms of plant-derived natural products in the treatment of cervical cancer. *Biomolecules* 11, 1539.

Jiang, J., Cao, D., Tsukamoto, T., Wang, G., Jia, Z., Suo, J., Cao, X. (2013). Anticancer effects of 4-vinyl-2,6-dimethoxyphenol (canolol) against SGC-7901 human gastric carcinoma cells. *Oncology Letters* 5, 1562–1566.

Klaunig, J. (2018). Oxidative stress and cancer. *Current Pharmaceutical Design* 24, 4771–4778.

Kolak, A., Kamińska, M., Sygit, K., Budny, A., Surdyka, D., Kukiełka-Budny, B., Burdan, F. (2017). Primary and secondary prevention of breast cancer: Annals of agricultural and environmental medicine. *AAEM* 24, 549–553.

Kraljić, K., Brkan, V., Skevin, D., Srcek, V. G., Radosevic, K. (2019). Canolol dimer, a biologically active phenolic compound of edible rapeseed oil. *Lipids* 54, 189–200.

Kuwahara, H., Kanazawa, A., Wakamatu, D., Morimura, S., Kida, K., Akaike, T., Maeda, H. (2004). Antioxidative and antimutagenic activities of 4-vinyl-2,6-dimethoxyphenol (canolol) isolated from canola oil. *Journal of Agricultural and Food Chemistry* 52, 4380–4387.

Llovet, J., Kelley, R., Villanueva, A., Singal, A., Pikarsky, E., Roayaie, S., Lencioni, R., Koike, K., Zucman-Rossi, J., Finn, R. (2021). Hepatocellular carcinoma. *Nature Reviews Disease Primers* 7, 1–28.

Maeda, H., Cao, X., Tsukamoto, T., Seki, T., Kuwahara, H., Tatematsu, M. (2006). Inhibition of bacterial mutagenesis and carcinogenesis in *Helicobacter pylori*-infected gerbil model by using a phenolic compound from crude rape seed oil, canolol. *Nitric Oxide* 14, 17.

Miller, K., Nogueira, L., Mariotto, A., Rowland, J., Yabroff, K., Alfano, C., Jemal, A., Kramer, J., Siegel, R. (2019). Cancer treatment and survivorship statistics, 2019. *CA: A Cancer Journal for Clinicians* 69, 363–385.

Montoya-Gómez, A., Montealegre-Sánchez, L., García-Perdomo, H., Jiménez-Charris, E. (2020). Cervical cancer and potential pharmacological treatment with snake venoms. *Molecular Biology Reports* 47, 4709–4721.

Seyed, M., Jantan, I., Bukhari, S., Vijayaraghavan, K. (2016). A comprehensive review on the chemotherapeutic potential of piceatannol for cancer treatment, with mechanistic insights. *Journal of Agricultural and Food Chemistry* 64, 725–737.

Siegel, R., Miller, K., Jemal, A. (2019) Cancer statistics. *CA: A Cancer Journal for Clinicians* 69, 7–34.

Smyth, E., Nilsson, M., Grabsch, H., van Grieken, N., Lordick, F. (2020). Gastric cancer. *Lancet (London, England)* 396, 635–648.

Xia, X., Xiang, X., Huang, F., Zheng, M., Zhang, Z., Han, L. (2019). Dietary canolol induces apoptosis in human cervical carcinoma HeLa cells through ROS-MAPK mediated mitochondrial signaling pathway: *In vitro and in vivo*. *Chemico-Biological Interactions* 300, 138–150.

Xu, Y., Jiang, F., Song, J., Yang, X., Shu, N., Yuan, L., Tan, C., Liu, Y. (2020). Understanding of the role of pretreatment methods on rapeseed oil from the perspective of phenolic compounds. *Journal of Agricultural and Food Chemistry* 68, 8847–8854.

Yang, W., Zeng, X., Liu, Z., Zhao, Q., Tan, Y., Gao, J., Li, H., Xiang, Y. (2020). Diet and liver cancer risk: A narrative review of epidemiological evidence. *British Journal of Nutrition* 124, 1–31.

Zhang, J., Li, L., Wang, Z., Zheng, C., Zhang, H., Wang, H., Li, P., Zhai, X., Li, H., Tan, X. (2017). Inhibitory mechanism against oxidative stress and bilogical activities of canolol. *Acta Poloniae Pharmaceutica* 74, 25–29.

chapter seven

Application of canolol in foods

Bertrand Matthäus, Michael N. A. Eskin, Ruchira Nandasiri, Maryam Nikbakht Nasrabadi, and Supratim Ghosh

7.1 Introduction

Today one of the most important problems in the supply of food to mankind is food waste. According to the United Nations Environment Program (UNEP) nearly 931 million tons of food are discarded worldwide, corresponding to 17% of total food production (United Nations Environment Programme 2021). That means that 112 kilograms of food are discarded per person per year on the consumer level, with nearly three quarters of it in the household. Overall, this is not economically nor socially or environmentally sustainable. Calculations show that as much as 8%–10% of global greenhouse gas emissions are caused by food that is not consumed (Mbow et al. 2019). Therefore, all measures that help to prevent food waste are also a contribution to environmental protection and the sustainability of food production.

A major contributor to food waste is oxidation, which leads to the deterioration of color, texture, nutrients, smell, and taste of food during storage, shortens the shelf life, and causes substantial economic losses (Barden and Decker 2016). In particular, the formation of off-flavor resulting from the degradation of fatty acids and proteins leads to lower acceptance by consumers and thus to food being rejected and disposed. However, lipid oxidation has not only adverse effect on food quality but also on human health. Uptake of potentially toxic lipid oxidation products through the diet have shown correlation with different inflammatory diseases as well as cancer, atherosclerosis, and aging (Vieira et al. 2017).

Important for preventing lipid oxidation in food are antioxidants that naturally occur in food or are added during food processing. In earlier years, these were mainly synthetic antioxidants such as BHT, BHA, or TBHQ, while today consumers prefer natural ones such as tocopherols, ß-carotene, or rosemary extract. In the last years canolol, also known as vinylsyringol or 2,6-dimethoxy-4-vinylphenol, came up as a very promising natural antioxidant isolated from heat-treated rapeseed as result from

DOI: 10.1201/b22828-7

decarboxlyation of sinapic acid. In this chapter the antioxidant activity of canolol in comparison to other synthetic and natural antioxidants as well as the application during food processing is shown.

7.2 Properties of canolol

Canolol is a phenolic compound formed during heating of rapeseed as a result of oilseed processing or roasting. The higher temperature results in decarboxylation of sinapic acid with release of carbon dioxide and loss of the carboxyl group. Thus, canolol has a vinyl group that extends the system of delocalized double bonds of the phenol ring of the molecule. In addition, the molecule comprises of two methoxyl ($-OCH_3$) and one phenolic hydroxyl (–OH) groups which can also promote the antioxidant activity (Chen et al. 2020). The high reactivity of the molecule in the presence of oxygen leads among others to dimers, trimers, and oligomers (Harbaum-Piayda et al. 2010; Nandasiri et al. 2021).

Due to the system of delocalized double bonds and the presence of methoxyl and hydroxyl groups, canolol shows a remarkable antioxidant activity and the ability to scavenge free radicals. This antioxidant and lipid protective activity have been described by Koski et al. (2003) as similar to that of γ-tocopherol. Wakamatsu et al. (2005) found the efficiency of canolol as an alkyl peroxyl radical scavenger better than that of α-tocopherol, vitamin C, β-carotene, rutin, or quercetin. The ß-carotene-linoleic acid assay determines the capability of an antioxidant to slow down the lipid peroxidation in the phase of initiation as well as in the phase of propagation (Marco 1968). This reaction is based on the co-oxidation of ß-carotene by oxidized linoleic acid and the resulting decolorization of ß-carotene that is influenced by the presence of antioxidants. The decolorization can be measured by UV spectroscopy at 417 nm. In this assay the effect of canolol is comparable to sinapic acid and slightly worse than for BHA or Trolox (Matthäus 2015).

The result showed (Figure 7.1) that the abstraction of the acid group from sinapic acid has no effect on the antioxidant activity of the resulting molecule in this assay. Due to the loss of the acid group canolol becomes significantly less polar than sinapic acid and may not be able to fully exhibit its antioxidant activity in the aqueous emulsion of linoleic acid and ß-carotene. Galano et al. (2011) showed the radical OOH scavenging activity of canolol is predicted to react about 3.6 times faster in lipid media than in aqueous solution with overall rate coefficients of 2.5×10^6 and $6.8 \times 10^5 M^{-1} s^{-1}$, respectively. They found similar activity to that of carotenes, higher than that of allicin, and much higher than that of melatonin. In the Rancimat test at 120°C and a constant air flow of 20 L/h canolol showed a positive effect on the oxidative stability of rapeseed oil. Pure rapeseed oil had a content of about 120 μg canolol/ g oil with an oxidative stability

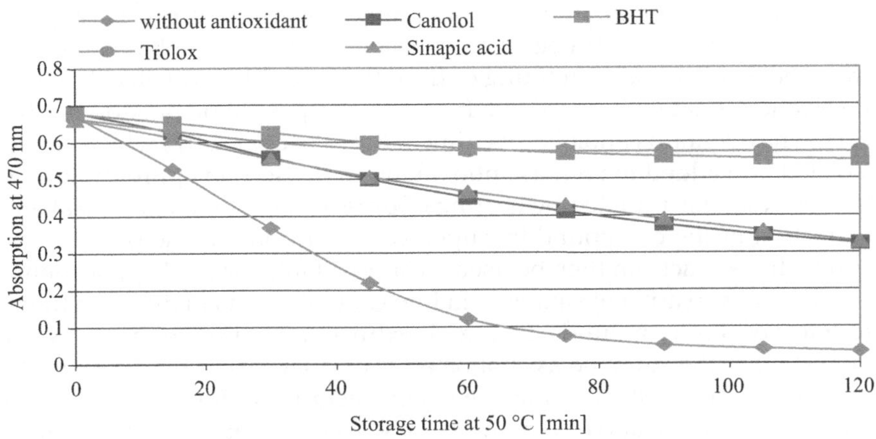

Figure 7.1 Purified canolol from oil of roasted rapeseeds: ß-carotene-linoleic acid assay.

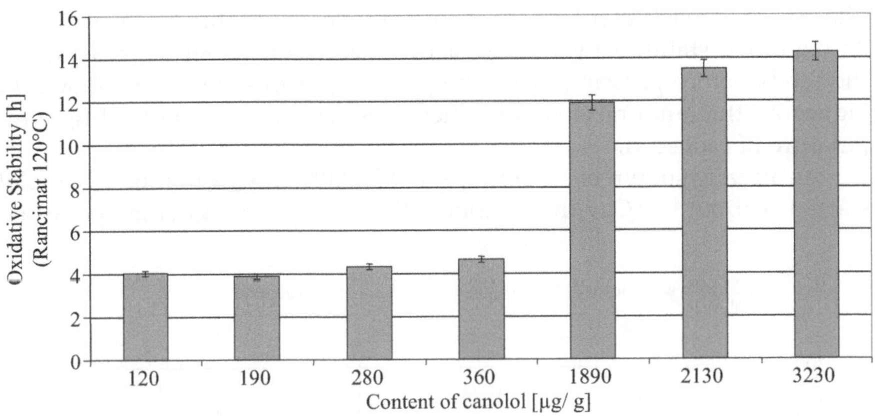

Figure 7.2 Influence of canolol content on oxidative stability in the Rancimat test.

in the Rancimat test of 4 h. With increasing amounts of canolol up to 3220 µg/g the oxidative stability increased more than 3-fold to about 14.2 h (Figure 7.2).

This high antioxidant activity of canolol makes the compound interesting for the application as stabilizer in food systems.

For the application of canolol in food two different approaches are conceivable. The first approach uses the intrinsic formation of canolol during heating or roasting of rapeseed and co-extraction of the compound together with the oil by screw-pressing or solvent extraction (Pudel et al. 2014). This may lead to an improved oxidative stability of the resulting rapeseed oil. To obtain canolol-containing extracts that can be applied to stabilize food two strategies are possible. They can be obtained either from the deodistillate of refining or from the by-products of oil extraction. If solvent-extracted oil is refined, fractions of rapeseed oil deodorizer distillate may contain canolol or its dimers (Oehlke et al. 2017) which can be isolated and added to food as antioxidant. In the second approach formation of canolol is initiated by heating of press cake or extraction meal and extraction of the compound by supercritical carbon dioxide (Pudel et al. 2014). This extract can then be used as antioxidants for food applications.

The conversation of sinapic acid into canolol results in different transfer rates of the compounds during oil extraction by a screw press. While almost all of the sinapine as choline ester of sinapic acid remained in the press cake, only 1.4%–2.7% of the sinapic acid was found. On the other hand between% 56 and 83% of the canolol was transferred to the oil (Yang et al. 2014).

7.3 *Intrinsic formation of canolol*

The first approach can be useful to improve oil quality with regard to its oxidative stability by means of oil processing either by roasting of the seeds before pressing or by the pressing process itself. As shown in Figure 7.3 the amount of canolol increases with increasing heating temperature of rapeseed.

As already shown by Spielmeyer et al. (2009), the formation of canolol started at about 160°C with an exponential increase at higher temperature.

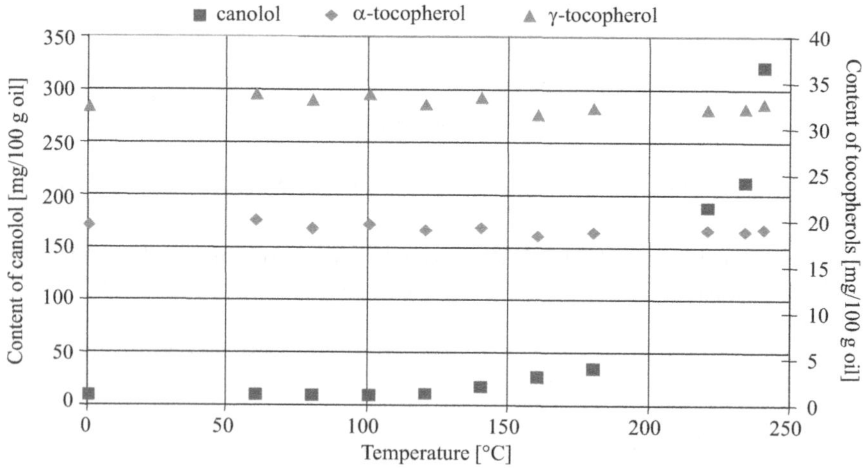

Figure 7.3 Influence of temperature during roasting on formation of canolol and content of tocopherols.

If this approach should be applied to the production of cold-pressed oils it has to be taken into consideration that at higher temperatures of roasting, flavor compounds from the Maillard reaction are formed that deeply change the sensory quality of the resulting oil from seed-like and nutty via roasting to burnt and bitter. In addition, the oil also gets a darker color from colored reaction products of the Maillard reaction (Tamanna and Mahmood 2015). Therefore, it is necessary and recommended to balance the heating time and temperature of the roasting process in such a way that, on the one hand, as much canolol as possible is formed and, on the other hand, the sensory quality of the oil is influenced as little as possible. Here a roasted taste and smell of the resulting oil is preferred. In addition, Spielmeyer et al. (2009) showed that the amount of canolol can be reduced during heat treatment by the reaction of canolol with other constituents of the rapeseed, such as lipid hydroperoxides formed during the heating. Also, a degradation of canolol by pyrolysis or thermal decomposition is possible. Oehlke et al. (2017) showed the formation of dimers, trimers, and oligomers by longer and intensive heating.

One interesting tool for heating of rapeseed is the use of a microwave that allows a constant and reliable energy transport to the rapeseed. Zheng et al. (2014) investigated the effect of microwave treatment of rapeseed on the oxidative stability of the resulting rapeseed oil in comparison to untreated cold-pressed rapeseed oil and rapeseed oil stabilized by tertiary butyl-hydroquinone (TBHQ). The results showed that microwave treatment lead to an increase of phenolic compounds and canolol. During storage parameters describing the oxidative state of the oils increased in the order rapeseed oil from microwave-treated rapeseed < cold-pressed rapeseed oil + TBHQ < cold-pressed rapeseed oil. Also, Rekas et al. (2017) found an increase in canolol by the use of microwave treatment to a 7- and 23-fold higher amount in comparison to oil from unheated dehulled and whole rapeseed, respectively, resulting in a higher oxidative stability and radical scavenging activity of the resulting oil. On the other hand, the treatment also led to a darkening of the oil. In this experiment, dehulling resulted in higher initial content of phenolic acids in oil from dehulled seeds, while the content of canolol was higher in oil from whole seeds. One explanation is the different pressing conditions of dehulled and whole seeds in the screw press resulting in higher amounts of canolol in oil from whole seeds due to a higher temperature during pressing as a result of the higher friction energy due to the hulls. The content of canolol showed a positive significant correlation with the induction period measured by the Rancimat test as $r = 0.996$ for oil from whole seeds and $r = 0.920$ for oil from dehulled seeds. However, Shrestha and de Meulenaer (2014) showed that mustard oil from roasted seeds had significantly higher oxidative stability than mustard oil from unroasted seeds fortified with an equivalent amount of canolol. Both oils showed a higher oxidative stability than oil from unroasted seeds, indicating the effect of canolol. From this they assumed that canolol formation as a result of roasting cannot fully explain the increasing oxidative stability of oils from roasted seeds. Higher extraction yields of phospholipids or Maillard reaction products are also responsible for the better stability.

Siger et al. (2016) demonstrated that roasting temperature between 140°C and 160°C resulted in less canolol in the resulting cold-pressed oil while at temperature of 180°C a stronger destruction of the cell structure occurred with the result that more canolol passed into the oil (609 μg/g at 180°C, 15 min). In this investigation the authors found an increasing amount of tocopherols in rapeseed oil obtained from heat-treated seeds at 180°C.

Another interesting approach to initiate the formation of canolol in rapeseed that can be co-extracted with the oil during oil processing is air-frying of rapeseed (Fadairo et al. 2023). The authors found a temperature-time association for the recovery of canolol and showed that the highest yield of canolol in the resulting oil was found at 190°C and 15 min. This oil also showed a greater in vitro antioxidant activity in different tests such as DPPH free radical scavenging ability or FRAP test with a strong positive correlation between canolol content to the antioxidative activities.

7.3.1 Canolol isolated from deodistillate

In crude rapeseed oil canolol is the predominant phenolic compound, accounting for about 85% of the total phenolic compounds (Kraljić et al. 2015). During the refining process of crude rapeseed oil different bioactive compounds such as tocopherols, phytosterols, carotinioids, phenolic copounds, and canolol are removed entirely or partially during the deodorization step together with other constituents, mainly free fatty acids, triacylglycerols, or contaminants. These compounds accumulate in the deodistillate as by-products of the refining process. Harbaum-Piayda et al. (2010) found 226 mg/kg canolol in the deodistillate while in refined rapeseed oil no canolol was detected. Virgin and steam-treated rapeseed oil with no further refining contained traces – 6.7 and 5.7–14.6 mg/kg canolol – showing that the compound is stripped from the rapeseed oil during deodorization. These results are in agreement with results from Spielmeyer et al. (2009), who found no canolol in refined rapeseed oil but amounts in the range from 9.3 to 81.4 mg/kg in five commercial cold-pressed rapeseed oils. In addition, the deodistillate comprised of high amounts of dimers and trimers of canolol (3479 and 3451 mg/kg, respectively). These compounds can also be found in refined rapeseed oil in amounts between traces and 46.5 mg/kg as well as traces and 63.0 mg/kg. Kraljić et al. (2015) demonstrated that the amount of canolol decreased during the subsequent refining steps, however on the other hand 4-vinylsyringol dimer appeared as a new compound formed from canolol during the processing. In the crude oil this compound is not present, but it is formed during neutralization and then steadily decreases during the further refining steps from 29.8 mg/kg after neutralization to 16.4 mg/kg after deodorization when canolol is almost removed. The authors also showed that the formation of the dimer occurs only under acidic conditions, probably via electrophilic aromatic substitution of 4-vinylsyringol. In the ORAC test using physiological relevant pH-values at 37°C canolol showed values of 17.8427 µM TE per mg while for the dimer a value of 84.0193 µM per mg was found (Kraljić et al. 2019).

In storage experiments with canolol and vinylsyringol dimer added to purified rapeseed oil triacylglycerols, Oehlke et al. (2017) showed the strong effect of the purified compounds to inhibit the formation of hydroperoxides, propanal, and hexanal during storage at 40°C in the dark. As expected, this protective effect was less pronounced during storage at 25°C in the light.

7.4 Deep-fat frying

Deep-fat frying is one of the most popular processes for the preparation of food. During the process the frying medium is exposed to heat, air, and water from the foods. These conditions result in the degradation of the frying medium and the formation of short-chain aroma-active compounds or di- and oligomers impairing oil and finally food quality. These degradation products not only influence the sensory quality but also the palatability and the shelf life of the food. One factor influencing the stability of frying oils is the presence of naturally present or added antioxidants that can decrease the oxidation during frying. Examples are tocopherols and rosemary extract as natural antioxidants or tert-butylhydroquinone (TBHQ) and butylated hydroxyanisole (BHA) as synthetic ones. Both types of antioxidants are more or less suitable to slow down oxidation, however at frying temperature the effectiveness of these antioxidants decreases or is no longer present due to losses through volatilization or decomposition (Boskou 1988; Choe and Min 2007).

In different frying experiments the strong effect of canolol to slow down the degradation of the frying medium has been shown (Aachary et al. 2014; Matthäus et al. 2014). Aachary et al. (2014) investigated the effect of crude canolol extracted from canola meal by accelerated solvent extraction and phenolic extracts from canola oil deodistillates for their potential to stabilize rapeseed oil during deep-fat frying in comparison to BHT. The results revealed significantly ($p < 0.05$) lower values for the total oxidation (TOTOX) and conjugated diene/triene values of oils stabilized with canolol extracts obtained from the deodistillate and from heat-treated rapeseed in comparison to BHT. Comparing both extracts of canolol showed a stronger effect of canolol extracted from heat-treated rapeseed on the different parameters describing the oxidative state of the frying medium. The authors assumed that a further purification of the extract from the deodistillate may improve the stabilizing effect of this extract. In summary they concluded that both canolol extracts are effective in inhibiting lipid oxidation during deep-fat frying.

Matthäus et al. (2014) used a canolol-enriched extract obtained from rapeseed meal heat-treated in a fluidized bed and extracted by super-critical carbon dioxide (Pudel et al. 2014). This extract mainly consisted of triacylglycerols (68.2%), diacylglycerols (11.3%), and free fatty acids (9.7%) but also contained about 3% canolol. In the frying experiment different amounts of the extract, calculated as 200, 500, and 750 mg/kg canolol were added to rapeseed oil and the frying performance was compared to rapeseed oil without added antioxidant as control and rapeseed oil fortified with 200 mg/kg TBHQ and rosemary extract (40 and 200 mg/kg), respectively. After 30 h of deep-fat frying canolol enriched rapeseed oils showed a two to three times better frying performance in comparison to the other oils with regards to the formation of di- and polymer triacylglycerols, total polar compounds, secondary degradation products (anisidine value) and iodine value. The experiment also showed a significant slower degradation of α- and γ-tocopherol. The authors calculated the LD50-values for α- and γ-tocopherol which indicates the time in which half of the tocopherols are degraded under frying conditions. While the LD50-values for the control, rosemary extract (40 and 200 mg/kg), and TBHQ were 5.4, 6.0, 8.5, and 4.6 h (α-tocopherol) and 5.8, 6.5, 8.3, and 5.0 h (γ-tocopherol), respectively, canolol showed a strong dose-dependent effect on stabilizing α-and γ-tocopherol in frying oils with 17.9, 23.6, and 28.7 h (α-tocopherol) and 15.8, 18.1, and 19.6 h (γ-tocopherol), respectively, for rapeseed oil fortified with 200, 500, and 750 mg/kg canolol (Figure 7.4).

This strong effect of canolol increases the service life of the tocopherols during deep-fat frying which may have a positive effect on the product being fried and its shelf-life.

Matthäus et al. (2014) also investigated the dependence of the canolol concentration in the frying oil on the effect of stabilization and the degradation rate of canolol during frying. The influence of canolol-enriched extract showed a strong concentration-dependent effect on the frying performance. At higher concentrations the stabilizing effect of the extract was higher. In addition, the degradation rate of canolol was decreased at higher concentration, with similar degradation rates for oils fortified with 500 and 750 mg/kg canolol (slope: −0.25 and −0.26, respectively), and a higher degradation rate for oil fortified with 200 mg/kg canolol (slope: −0.47). The authors assumed that canolol may have a role in stabilizing itself during frying.

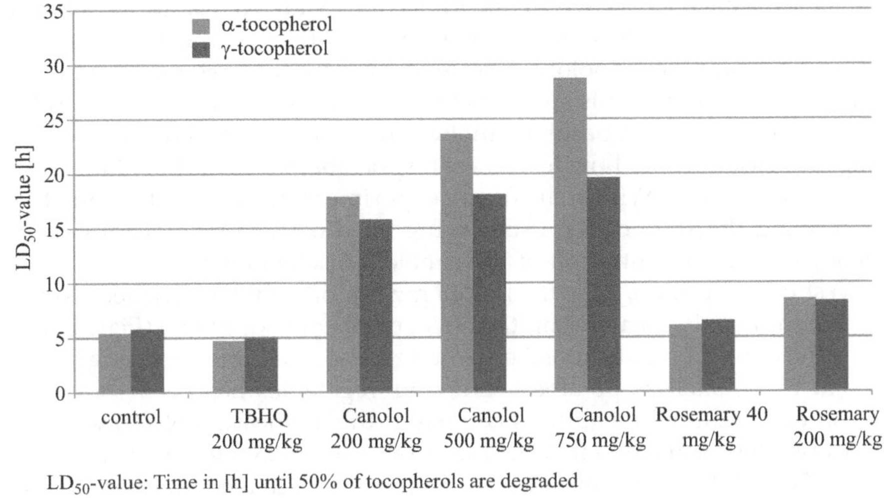

Figure 7.4 Effect of canolol on the degradation of tocopherols in a frying medium.

As a clear drawback of the use of canolol extracted by super-critical carbon dioxide from heat-treated rapeseed, the authors have noted that the addition of the extract resulted in higher initial acid values of the frying media due to the high concentration of free fatty acids in the extract. In particular, when larger amounts of canolol were added it is possible that the limit for free fatty acids defined in different countries as parameter for discarding the used frying medium can be reached. A further purification of such extracts seems to be necessary and can avoid this problem if free fatty acids are removed. According to the authors it is also not clear whether the stabilizing effect of the extract only results from canolol or also from other co-extracted compounds. For example, it is known that constituents such as phospholipids or Maillard reaction products formed during roasting or hot pressing could also improve the oxidative stability (Shrestha and de Meulenaer, 2014). In summary, the authors stated that canolol is a very strong antioxidant that can be used to improve the thermal stability of frying oils remarkably.

In a simulated frying experiment Matthäus et al. (2015) investigated the effect of pure canolol in comparison to an enriched canolol extract obtained by fluidized bed treatment. They compared the effect of different lower concentrations of the extract with TBHQ. The principle of the experiment was that the oils fortified with antioxidants were heated at 170°C over a period of 8 h in an apparatus similar to the Rancimat with an air flow of 20 L/h. For each sample 100 g of oil was weighted into an appropriate glass tube. The results for total polar compounds, di- and oligomer triacylglycerols, and anisidine value showed a significant lower increase for all antioxidants in comparison to the control. The strongest effect was found for canolol extract even in comparison to pure canolol in equimolar amounts. This supports the assumption from Shrestha and De Meulenaer (2014) that besides canolol other constituents co-extracted by super-critical carbon dioxide also are responsible for the antioxidant effect of canolol extracts. Within the frying experiment the different parameters describing the state of the used frying oil showed a significant dependency on the concentration of the canolol enriched extracts. Even at the lowest concentration, the effect of 25 mg/kg oil canolol enriched extract was significantly greater than the effect of 200 mg/kg TBHQ (Figure 7.5).

The application of canolol enriched rapeseed oil for stir-frying of different foods such as potatoes, tofu, and vegetables has been shown by Zhou et al. (2019). The authors compared the application of rapeseed oil with two levels of canolol (528.9 mg/kg versus 250.5 mg/kg). The formation of canolol was achieved by heating rapeseed in a commercial tunnel microwave oven (2,459 Hz, 55 KW) for 7 min. The high canolol rapeseed oil showed a better stir-frying performance with regard to the peroxide value, anisidine value, and malondialdehyde as parameters describing the oxidation state of the used oils. Stir-frying showed significant losses of canolol during processing with 55%–64.5% for high canolol rapeseed oil and canolol contents in the range of 187.8–237.7 mg/kg after processing, and losses of 61.5%–81.8% for low canolol rapeseed oil with canolol levels in the range of 45.6–96.4 mg/kg, respectively. The content of α- and

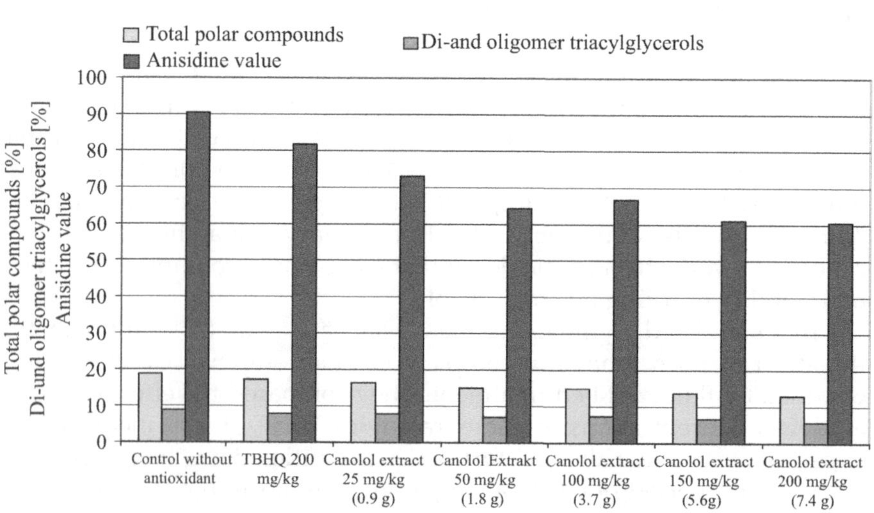

Figure 7.5 Comparison between different amounts of canolol extract in a simulated frying experiment.

γ-tocopherols in high canolol rapeseed oil was significantly higher than those in low canolol rapeseed oil. The authors concluded that the presence of higher amounts of canolol would be advantageous for stir-frying.

In China, so-called fragrant rapeseed oil has become increasingly popular because of its unique flavor. The Chinese standard defines this type of oil as cold-pressed rapeseed oil obtained from roasted seeds without the addition of other spices. In a frying experiment, Cao et al. (2023) added different amounts of phenolic extracts obtained from rapeseed oil by extraction with 70% methanol.

The authors showed that high-canolol phenolic extracts significantly inhibited the increase in peroxide, acid value, *p*-anisidine value, and carbonyl values, as well as total polar compounds and degradation of unsaturated fatty acids in fragrant rapeseed oil during frying over 24 h. In addition, the high-canolol phenolic extract significantly reduced the formation of compounds responsible for the off-flavor of frying oil (hexanoic acid, nonanoic acid, etc.). On the other hand, the extract inhibited the degradation of some typical deep-fat frying flavor compounds such as (E,E)-2,4-decadienal.

The sensory evaluation of the used frying oils with and without high-canolol phenolic extract revealed no significant effect on the typical attributes of fragrant rapeseed oil such as pungent, grassy, and nutty. But the addition of extract resulted in a positive effect on the deep-fried flavor which was stabilized by the inhibition of the rancid flavour. From these results they concluded that the application of high-canolol phenolic extracts is able to protect the quality of fragrant rapeseed oil and to prolong its shelf life during storage.

7.5 Lipid oxidation in emulsions

An emulsion is a colloidal dispersion consisting of two immiscible liquids, typically one being water and the other oil or fat, stabilized by a surface-active agent. In an emulsion, tiny droplets of one liquid are dispersed throughout the other. The emulsifying agent or emulsifier helps to prevent the droplets from coalescing or separating, allowing for the creation of a stable colloidal system. Emulsions are commonly used in various aspects of daily life. They are widely used in the food industry for products like salad dressings, mayonnaise, cream-based sauces, and beverages as well as in cosmetics, pharmaceuticals, and many other industries (McClements 2015). Emulsions are widely used in food formulations as a delivery system for functional and bioactive lipids such as polyunsaturated fatty acids (PUFAs), making them susceptible to lipid oxidation. Omega-3 fatty acids, such as eicosapentaenoic acid (EPA) and docosahexaenoic acid (DHA), are well-known for their health benefits, including cardiovascular protection, brain health and development, lowering blood pressure, and anti-inflammatory effects (Kapoor et al. 2021). Incorporating omega-3 oils into emulsions offers a convenient way to deliver these essential fatty acids to consumers. Emulsions can boost the bioavailability of omega-3 oils, as the micro- or nano-sized lipid droplets are readily digested and absorbed in the gastrointestinal tract after ingestion. Emulsifying omega-3 oils also facilitates their integration into aqueous-based food and beverage systems, thus broadening their applicability in a variety of product formulations. Additionally, the encapsulation of omega-3 oils in emulsions allows for the incorporation of other beneficial compounds or antioxidants, further enhancing the nutritional profile and oxidative stability of the end product. Thus, utilizing emulsions as a delivery system for omega-3 oils presents a promising approach to maximize both their functional benefits in food products and their health benefits for consumers. This makes emulsions appropriate for delivering omega-3 fatty acids in functional foods and dietary supplements. However, lipid oxidation is a significant concern in the application of omega-3-incorporated emulsions in the food and pharmaceutical industry, as it leads to the development of off-flavors, decreased nutritional value, and potential health risks associated with the consumption of oxidized lipids (Walker et al. 2015).

The nature of emulsions increases the susceptibility of lipids to oxidation. Due to the large interfacial area between the water and oil phases, more lipid molecules are exposed to pro-oxidative agents, such as light, heat, and metal ions (Villeneuve et al., 2021, Nasrabadi et al., 2019). The emulsifier present at the oil droplet surface can also promote or inhibit the interfacial lipid oxidation, depending on its properties and by changing the accessibility of reactants to the lipid phase (Villeneuve et al., 2021, Nasrabadi 2019). Furthermore, the presence of water and oxygen emulsions provides an environment conducive to the formation of various reactive oxygen species (ROS), which are key players in lipid oxidation (Villeneuve et al., 2021). In bulk oil, lipid oxidation predominantly occurs in a more homogeneous phase, and the rate is mainly influenced by the type of fatty acids, various minor components, moisture, and other pro- and anti-oxidants (Mohanan et al., 2018; Laguerre et al., 2015). In contrast, in emulsions, oxidation is more complex due to the heterogeneous nature and increased surface area of the lipid phase. Consequently, an antioxidant's effectiveness in emulsions hinges significantly on its position at the interface, influenced by its polarity. These differences often lead to a faster oxidation rate in emulsions than in bulk oils (Villeneuve et al. 2021).

Several strategies have been employed for the prevention of lipid oxidation in emulsions. Since in oil-in-water (O/W) emulsions oxidation primarily occurs at the interface where PUFAs from the oil phase interact with pro-oxidants in the water phase, the composition, thickness, and charge of the interface can be designed to minimize the exposure of lipids to pro-oxidative agents (Laguerre et al. 2015). As the interface becomes thicker and stronger using proteins and protein-polysaccharide complexes and conjugates, the emulsion would be more stable against oxidation. For instance, Nasrabadi et al. (2019) found that flaxseed O/W emulsion stabilized by flaxseed protein-flaxseed mucilage complexes experienced slower oxidation compared to those using only flaxseed protein and polysorbate 80, which is a small molecule surfactant. Applying metal chelators or stabilizers and emulsifiers with metal ion–binding ability can also reduce their catalytic effect in the oxidation process (Haahr and Jacobsen, 2008).

The most common strategy to prevent lipid oxidation in emulsion is using antioxidants to scavenge free radicals. Synthetic antioxidants, such as BHT, BHA, and TBHQ, have been widely used; however, consumer demand toward the use of more natural food ingredients has led to the search for an effective natural antioxidant (Shahidi and Ambigaipalan, 2015). Canolol, has shown promising effects as an antioxidant in emulsions due to its ability to scavenge free radicals by the transfer of hydrogen atoms from their phenolic moiety (Galano et al. 2011). This, combined with its ability to integrate into the emulsion interface, makes it particularly effective in protecting against lipid oxidation. Table 7.1 summarizes the results of utilization of various canola and mustard extracts to prevent lipid oxidation in O/W emulsions. Sørensen et al. (2013) compared the antioxidant ability of canolol, sinapic acid, and sinapine extracts obtained from canola meal for canola O/W emulsions and compared their ability to prevent lipid oxidation against BHT. According to their findings, at 350 mM, canolol showed the highest antioxidant activity after BHT. The authors proposed that the difference in antioxidant abilities between

Table 7.1 Summary of literature on the utilization of various canola and mustard extracts in preventing lipid oxidation in oil-in-water (O/W) emulsions

Extract type	Oil	Major findings	References
Canolol, sinapic acid and sinapine extracts obtained from canola meal	Canola O/W emulsion	Compared separately with BHT, at 350 mM, canolol showed the highest antioxidant activity after BHT.	Sørensen et al. (2013)
Canolol	Tuna O/W emulsion	Fortification of tuna oil could improve the oxidative stability of emulsions.	Logan and Fagan (2013)

(*Continued*)

Table 7.1 (Continued)

Extract type	Oil	Major findings	References
Sinapic acid derivatives: syringic acid, syringaldehyde, sinapine, canolol, and ethyl, propyl, and butyl sinapate	Sunflower O/W emulsion, liposome suspension, and oleogel	Sinapic acid esters (ethyl, propyl, and butyl sinapate) showed the highest antioxidant ability in the emulsion and liposome while syringic acid and syringaldehyde showed the best performance in bulk oil due to higer polarity. Canolol showed higher ability in oleogel.	Martinović et al. (2019)
White mustard seed extract containing canolol, *p*-hydroxybenzoic and sinapic acids	Sunflower O/W emulsion, bulk oil, and oleogel	Oxidation prevention in emulsion by the mustard seed extract was comparable to that of Trolox, but less than half that of BHT. In bulk oil, both the extract and Trolox had superior antioxidant effect than BHT.	Martinović et al. (2020)
Phenolic-rich mustard extract	Flaxseed O/W emulsion	The incorporation of extract was successful in depressing the formation of oxidation products at 4, 25 and 60°C during 28 days of storage. Results were comparable to TBHQ.	Nasrabadi et al. (unpublished)

canolol, sinapic acid, and sinapine is not solely based on their capacity to scavenge free radicals but is also significantly influenced by their polarity, leading to different locations in the emulsions. As mentioned before, the lipid oxidation in an emulsion initiates at the interface, and the ability of an antioxidant in localization at the interface determines its efficiency. Logan and Fagan (2013) also looked into the incorporation of canolol into the 10% w/w tuna O/W emulsion to improve its oxidative stability.

Martinović et al. (2019) compared different sinapic acid derivatives, including syringic acid, syringaldehyde, sinapine, canolol (4-vinylsyringol), and ethyl, propyl, and butyl sinapate, as well as BHT, as antioxidants in 10% w/w sunflower O/W emulsion as well as in bulk oil, liposome suspension, and oleogel. According to their results, sinapic acid esters, including ethyl, propyl, and butyl sinapate, showed the highest antioxidant ability in the emulsion and liposome suspension. However, in bulk oil, the more polar sinapic acid, syringic acid, and syringaldehyde showed the best performance. Canolol and butyl sinapate, which are less polar, displayed higher activity in oleogels due to their potential interactions with oil structuring agents. BHT proved more potent in preventing lipid oxidation in O/W emulsions than sinapic acid, canolol, and Trolox. However, in the context of bulk oil, sinapic acid, canolol, and Trolox performed better than BHT. These findings align with the polar paradox theory, which emphasizes the role of the lipid–water interfaces and surfaces in lipid peroxidation within mixed systems. The polar paradox suggests that in O/W emulsions, nonpolar antioxidants are more effective, while in bulk oils, polar antioxidants prevail. This observation shows the polar characteristics of the primary antioxidant components found in mustard seed extract, as described by Laguerre et al. (2015).

There are also some studies on the application of mustard or canola extracts containing a mixture of sinapic acid and its derivatives with a considerable amount of canolol for retarding lipid oxidation in emulsions. For instance, Martinović et al. (2020) reported that the antioxidant activity of mustard seed extract, containing high amounts of canolol and other sinapic acid derivatives, in sunflower O/W emulsion was comparable to that of Trolox.

While canolol shows promise as an antioxidant in emulsions, challenges remain. Its degree of polarity, solubility in vegetable oils, concentration, interaction with other food components, and stability during processing need further investigation. There's also a need to compare its efficacy with other antioxidants in complex food matrices. As consumers demand more natural and healthier products, canolol's potential use in emulsions holds significant promise for the future of food science. However, there remains a surprising dearth of comprehensive research focusing on its specific use in emulsions. The majority of existing studies have emphasized its antioxidant properties in bulk oils or other food systems, yet its interaction and effectiveness within emulsions remain under-explored. Emulsions present unique challenges due to the interface between oil and water phases, which necessitates specialized antioxidant mechanisms. Given canolol's promising antioxidant capabilities in other contexts, it is imperative to bridge this research gap. Such studies would not only enhance our understanding of canolol's range of applications but also potentially lead to innovative solutions for extending the shelf life and improving the quality of emulsified food products, particularly those containing sensitive lipids like omega-3 fatty acids. Future research might delve deeper into its application in diverse food systems and explore potential synergies with other natural antioxidants. Understanding the challenges and future perspectives in this field is essential for advancing the application of canolol and other antioxidants in emulsions.

7.6 Legal regulation

In the search for suitable and natural substances for the improvement of food quality, more and more compounds are being found, which, however, may not be used so easily. In most countries new food additives must be tested for their safety and only then may they be approved. The use of food additives is only allowed if there is a technological need and improvement of food quality. In Europe, the basis are regulation (EU) No. 1333/2008, regulation (EU) No. 1129/2011 and further amending regulations. In regulation (EC) No. 1129/2011, a list of compounds is presented that only are allowed as additives in food under the envisaged conditions of use. In order to get a new compound in this list, it is necessary to undergo an authorization process governed by regulation (EC) No. 1331/2008, which is based on the scientific risk assessment performed by the European Food Safety Authority (EFSA). EFSA has the duty to advise the European Commission, the European Parliament and EU Member States as risk managers in a strictly science-based advisory function.

Due to the antioxidant effect of the canolol extracts and their application for a specific technological reason, they belong to the food additives that have to be authorized before use in foods by EU legislation. For this all scientific data concerning application and safety has to be applied before EFSA will be asked for the scientific opinion. This process is time-consuming and costly but feasible for extracts with an added value.

References

Aachary, A. A., Chen, Y., Eskin, N. A. M., Thiyam-Hollander, U. (2014) Crude canolol and canola distillate extracts improve the stability of refined canola oil during deep-fat frying. *Eur J Lipid Sci Technol* 116, 1467–1476.

Barden, L., Decker, E. A. (2016) Lipid oxidation in low-moisture food: A review. *Crit Rev Food Sci Nutr* 56, 2467–2482.

Boskou, D. (1988) Stability of frying oils. G. Varela, A. E. Bender and I. D. Morton (Hg.): *Frying of food: Principles, changes, new approaches*. New York: VCH Publishers Ltd., S. 174–182.

Cao, L. L., Jia, P. P., Liu, H. T., Kang, S. M., Jiang, S. T., Pang, M. (2023) Effects of high-canolol phenolic extracts on fragrant rapeseed oil quality and flavor compounds during frying. *Foods* 12, 827.

Chen, J., Yang, J., Ma, L., Li, J., Shahzad, N., Kim, C. K. (2020) Structure-antioxidant activity relationship of methoxy, phenolic hydroxyl, and carboxylic acid groups of phenolic acids. *Scient Rep* 10, 2611.

Choe, E., Min, D. B. (2007) Chemistry of deep-fat frying oils. *J Food Sci* 72, R77–R86.

Fadairo, O. S., Nandasiri, R., Eskin, N. A. M., Aluko, R. E., Scanlon, M. G. (2023) Air frying as a heat pre-treatment method for improving the extraction and yield of canolol from canola seed oil. *Food Bioprocess Technol* 16, 639–651.

Galano, A., Francisco-Marquez, M., Alvarez-Idaboy, J. R. (2011) Canolol: A promising chemical agent against oxidative stress. *J Phys Chem B* 115, 8590–8596.

Haahr, A.-M., Jacobsen, C. (2008), Emulsifier type, metal chelation and pH affect oxidative stability of n-3-enriched emulsions. *Eur J Lipid Sci Technol*, 110, 949–961.

Harbaum-Piayda, B., Oehlke, K., Sönnichsen, F. D., Zacchi, P., Eggers, R., Schwarz, K. (2010) New polyphenolic compounds in commercial deodistillate and rapeseed oil. *Food Chem* 123, 607–615.

Kapoor, B., Kapoor, D., Gautam, S., Singh, R., Bhardwaj, S. (2021). Dietary polyunsaturated fatty acids (PUFAs): Uses and potential health benefits. *Curr Nutr Rep*, 10, 232–242.

Koski, A., Pekkarinen, S., Hopia, A., Wähälä, K., Heinonen, M. (2003) Processing of rapeseed oil. Effects on sinapinic acid derivative content and oxidative stability. *Eur Food Res Technol* 217, S. 110–114.

Kraljić, K., Brkan, V., Škevin, D., Srček, V. G., Radošević, K. (2019) Canolol dimer, a biologically active phenolic compound of edible rapeseed oil. *Lipids* 54, 189–200.

Kraljić, K., Skevin, D., Barisic, L., Kovacevic, M., Obranovic, M., Jurcevic, I. (2015) Changes in 4-vinylsyringol and other phenolics during rapeseed oil refining. *Food Chem* 187, 236–242.

Laguerre, M., Bayrasy, C., Panya, A., Weiss, J., McClements, D. J., Lecomte, J., Villeneuve, P. (2015) What makes good antioxidants in lipid-based systems? The next theories beyond the polar paradox. *Crit Rev Food Sci. Nutr*, 55, 183–201.

Logan, A., Fagan, P. (2013). Strategies to prevent oxidative deterioration in oil-in-water emulsion systems: Canola-based phenolic applications. In *Lipid Oxidation* Challenges in Food Systems, Editors: Logan, A., Nienaber, U., Pan, P., AOCS Press, Chapter 15, pp. 457–483, ISBN 9780983079163.

Marco, G. J. (1968) A rapid method for evaluation of antioxidants. *J Amer Oil Chem Soc* 45, 594–598.

Martinović, N., Polak, T., Ulrih, N. P., Abramovič, H. (2020). Mustard seed: Phenolic composition and effects on lipid oxidation in oil, oil-in-water emulsion and oleogel. *Ind Crop Prod*, 156, 112851.

Martinović, N., Ulrih, N. P., Abramovič, H. (2019), Sinapic acid and its derivatives increase oxidative stability in different model lipid systems. *Eur J Lipid Sci Technol*, 121, 1800326.

Matthäus, B., Chen, Y., Pudel, F., Achary, A., Thiyam-Holländer U. (2015) Application of canolol enriched extract from fluidized bed treated rapeseed meal as natural antioxidant in food processing. *13th Euro Fed Lipid Congress: Euro Fed Lipid. Florence,* Italy 27–30 September 2015.

Matthäus, B., Pudel, F., Chen, Y. G., Achary, A., Thiyam-Hollander, U. (2014) Impact of canolol-enriched extract from heat-treated canola meal to enhance oil quality parameters in deep-frying: A comparison with rosemary extract and TBHQ-fortified oil systems. *J Amer Oil Chem Soc* 91, 2065–2076.

Mbow, C., Rosenzweig, C., Barioni, L. G., Benton, T. G., Herrero, M., Krishnapillai, M., Liwenga E., Pradhan, P., Rivera-Ferre, M.G., Sapkota, T., Tubiello, F. N., Xu, Y. (2019). *Food Security Supplementary Material. In: Climate Change and Land: An IPCC special report on climate change, desertification, land degradation, sustainable land management, food security, and greenhouse gas fluxes in terrestrial ecosystems* [P.R. Shukla, J. Skea, E. Calvo Buendia, V. Masson-Delmotte, H.-O. Pörtner, D.C. Roberts, P. Zhai, R. Slade, S. Connors, R. van Diemen, M. Ferrat, E. Haughey, S. Luz, S. Neogi, M. Pathak, J. Petzold, J. Portugal Pereira, P. Vyas, E. Huntley, K. Kissick, M. Belkacemi, J. Malley, (eds.)]. Cambridge University Press, Cambridge, UK and New York, NY, USA, 896 pp. https://doi.org/10.1017/9781009157988

McClements, D. J. (2015). *Food Emulsions: Principles, Practices, and Techniques.* Third Edition (3rd ed.). CRC Press. https://doi.org/10.1201/b18868

Mohanan, A., Nickerson, M. T., Ghosh, S. (2018). Oxidative stability of flaxseed oil: Effect of hydrophilic, hydrophobic and intermediate polarity antioxidants. *Food Chem,* 266, 524–533.

Nandasiri, R., Imran, A., Thiyam-Hollander, U., Eskin, N. A.M. (2021) Rapidoxy (R) 100: A solvent-free pre-treatment for production of canolol. *Front Nutr* 8, 687851.

Nasrabadi, M. N., Hossein Goli, S. A., Dost A. S., Dewettinck, K., van der Meeren, P. (2019). Bioparticles of flaxseed protein and mucilage enhance the physical and oxidative stability of flaxseed oil emulsions as a potential natural alternative for synthetic surfactants. *Colloids Surf B: B,* 184, 110489.

Nasrabadi, M. N., Nandasiri, R., Thiyam-Hollander, U., Eskin, M., Ghosh, S. Phenolic-rich mustard extract significantly improved the oxidative stability of acidic pea protein-based flaxseed oil emulsions (unpublished)

Oehlke, K., Harbaum-Piayda, B., Meyer, F., Eggers, R., Schwarz, K. (2017) Antioxidant activity of deodorizer distillate fractions in rapeseed oil. *Eur J Lipid Sci Technol* 119 (7), 1600273.

Pudel, F., Habicht, V., Piofczyk, T., Matthäus, B., Quirin, K. W., Cawelius, A. (2014) Fluidized bed treatment of rapeseed meal and cake as possibility for the production of canolol. *OCL Oils Fat Crop Li* 21, D103.

Rekas, A., Siger, A., Wroniak, M., Scibisz, I., Derewiaka, D., Anders, A. (2017) Dehulling and microwave pretreatment effects on the physicochemical composition and antioxidant capacity of virgin rapeseed oil. *J Food Sci Technol-Mysore* 54, 627–638.

Shahidi, F., Ambigaipalan, P. (2015). Phenolics and polyphenolics in foods, beverages and spices: Antioxidant activity and health effects: A review. *J Funct Foods* 18, 820–897.

Shrestha, K., de Meulenaer, B. (2014) Effect of seed roasting on canolol, tocopherol, and phospholipid contents, maillard type reactions, and oxidative stability of mustard and rapeseed oils. *J Agr Food Chem* 62, S. 5412–5419.

Siger, A., Michalak, M., Rudzińska, M. (2016) Canolol, tocopherols, plastochromanol-8, and phytosterols content in residual oil extracted from rapeseed expeller cake obtained from roasted seed. *Eur J Lipid Sci Tech* 118, 1358–1367.

Sørensen, A. D. M., Friel, J., Winkler-Moser, J. K., Jacobsen, C., Huidrom, D., Reddy, N., Thiyam-Holländer, U. (2013). Impact of endogenous canola phenolics on the oxidative stability of oil-in-water emulsions. *Europ J Lip Sci Technol*, 115, 501–512.

Spielmeyer, A., Wagner, A., Jahreis, G. (2009) Influence of thermal treatment of rapeseed on the canolol content. *Food Chem* 112, 944–948.

Tamanna, N., Mahmood, N. (2015) Food processing and maillard reaction products: Effect on human health and nutrition. *Int J Food Sci*, 2015, 526762.

United Nations Environment Programme (2021) Food Waste Index Report 2021. Nairobi. 2021. United Nations Environment Programme. Nairobi. Online verfügbar unter https://www.unep.org/resources/report/unep-food-waste-index-report-2021,zuletztgeprüft am 27.04.2025.

Vieira, S. A., Zhang, G., Decker, E. A. (2017) Biological implications of lipid oxidation products. *J Am Oil Chem Soc* 94, 339–351.

Villeneuve, P., Bourlieu-Lacanal, C., Durand, E., Lecomte J., McClements, D. J., Decker, E. A. (2021) Lipid oxidation in emulsions and bulk oils: A review of the importance of micelles, *Crit Rev Food Sci Nutr*, 63, 4687–4727.

Wakamatsu, D., Morimura, S., Sawa, T., Kida, K., Nakai, C., Maeda, H. (2005) Isolation, identification, and structure of a potent alkyl-peroxyl radical scavenger in crude canola oil, canolol. *Biosci Biotech Bioch* 69, 1568–1574.

Walker, R., Decker, E. A., McClements, D. J. (2015). Development of food-grade nanoemulsions and emulsions for delivery of omega-3 fatty acids: Opportunities and obstacles in the food industry. *Food Function* 6, 41–54

Yang, M., Zheng, C., Zhou, Q., Liu, C. S., Li, W. L., Huang, F. H. (2014) Influence of microwaves treatment of rapeseed on phenolic compounds and canolol content. *J Agr Food Chem* 62, 1956–1963.

Zheng, C., Yang, M., Zhou, Q., Liu, C.-S., Huang, F.-H. (2014) Changes in the content of canolol and total phenolics, oxidative stability of rapeseed oil during accelerated storage. *Eur J Lipid Sci Technol* 116, 1675–1684.

Zhou, Q., Jia, X., Deng, Q., Chen, H., Tang, H., Huang, F. (2019) Quality evaluation of rapeseed oil in Chinese traditional stir-frying. *Food Sci Nutr* 7, 3731–3741.

Index

Pages in *italics* refer to figures

For Product Safety Concerns and Information please contact our
EU representative GPSR@taylorandfrancis.com Taylor & Francis
Verlag GmbH, Kaufingerstraße 24, 80331 München, Germany